Someone I LOVE is Dying

A Practical Guide for Honouring a Loved One Before and After Death

JEANNE M. SEDUN

Heart in Hand
BOOKS LTD.

Website: www.heartinhandbooks.com

Email: info@heartinhandbooks.com

Library and Archives Canada Cataloguing in Publication

Sedun, Jeanne M., author

Someone I love is dying : a practical guide for honouring a loved one before and after death / Jeanne M. Sedun.

Includes bibliographical references and index.
ISBN 978-0-9958178-0-7 (softcover)

1. Death--Psychological aspects. 2. Terminally ill--Psychology. 3. Death--Handbooks, manuals, etc. I. Title.

BF789.D4S38 2017 155.9'37 C2017-900878-1

Note: The information contained in this book is for general guidance only and was accurate at the time of writing. The contents of this book are not intended as a substitute for medical, legal, accounting or other professional advice. This book provides general information on the subject matter covered. Readers are encouraged to seek the services of a competent professional to discuss their own unique circumstances.

The author and publisher specifically disclaim any and all liability arising directly or indirectly from the use or application of any information contained in this book.

Special discounts are available on bulk purchases of this book for educational training purposes, fund-raising, or gift giving. Special editions or book excerpts can also be created to fit your specific needs. For information, please contact Heart in Hand Books Ltd. at info@heartinhandbooks.com.

Production Credits

Cover design by Carol Hyland, CS Creative

Book interior design / layout by Simon Troop, CS Creative

Printed and bound in Canada by Printorium Bookworks

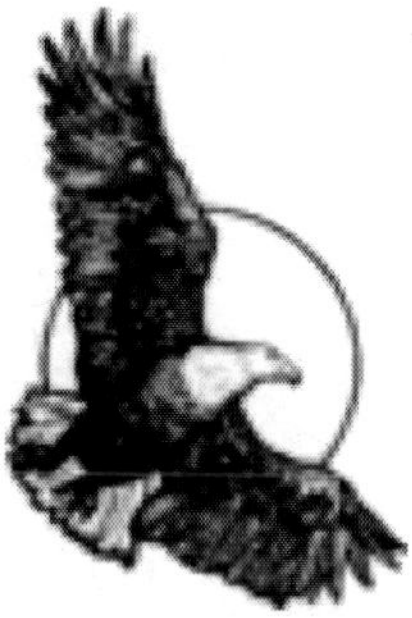

Dedication

Dedicated with love to "Grandma Rita"
– my mother and my friend.
Now that your suffering is over, may you
soar with eagles' wings.

ACKNOWLEDGMENTS

I want to thank the following people without whom this book would not have been possible:

- My mother, Rita Mae, who inspired me to write this book. I miss your friendship and your presence in my life.
- My husband and my best friend Thom. You supported me through my mother's illness and death – one of the most difficult experiences I have ever gone through. Thank you for loving me, and for giving me the time and freedom to travel to Quadra Island to write this book in honour of my mother.
- My beautiful children Samuel and Geneviève. You are part of Grandma Rita's legacy. I am so very proud of you. Your tender and caring hearts would make Grandma Rita proud.
- My friend Faye Schmidt, for sharing her suggestions and experiences while caring for her ailing mother, and for her encouragement to publish this book.
- My friend Lloyd Duhaime, for his legal expertise, quirky sense of humour, and courage in the face of adversity.
- Victoria Hospice, who cared for my mother in her final days.

ABOUT THE AUTHOR

Jeanne Sedun is an Executive Director with the Government of British Columbia where she has served for more than two decades. She holds degrees in arts and education from the University of Winnipeg, where she was a silver medal winner, and a Master of Divinity Degree from the Canadian Southern Baptist Seminary.

Jeanne has a unique combination of practical writing and communication skills, the ability to challenge and inspire, and compassion for others. Drawing on her training as a teacher, project manager and Protestant minister, she creates a roadmap for supporting a loved one facing a terminal illness. She has two adult children and lives in Victoria, British Columbia with her husband. Jeanne is fluent in French, and in her spare time enjoys swimming, learning about wine and travel. She is a harp student at the Victoria Conservatory of Music.

FOR INFORMATION

Requests for further information, as well as inquiries about the author's availability for book signing events and speaking engagements should be directed to the address below. Readers of this book are also encouraged to contact the author with comments and ideas for future editions.

Email: info@heartinhandbooks.com

Website: www.heartinhandbooks.com

Facebook: www.facebook.com/HeartinHandBooks

WHAT PEOPLE ARE SAYING ABOUT

Someone I Love is Dying

"For many, supporting someone through their end of life journey means travelling with them on a difficult, twisting road that is poorly marked. On this road our usual driving and navigation skills can easily fall short. At long last, Jeanne Sedun has created a guide for this journey that illuminates the road in very practical ways. Her book Someone I Love is Dying *fills the void of information by clearly laying out what needs to be done as this journey is made. It is a must read for everyone supporting a loved one at the end of their life."*

Faye Schmidt, family member who supported a loved one and who wishes this book had been available then

"If you've ever had to face the potentially terminal illness of a parent or other loved one, you will know how challenging it is to manage the many pressing practical issues even while you are grappling with powerful emotional ones. Anyone who finds themselves in this place will find enormous comfort and practical guidance in Someone I Love is Dying.

Jeanne Sedun treats this difficult subject with honesty, sensitivity and clarity. She provides examples, checklists and forms to guide the reader through tasks they will need to face, and in so doing eases the way. This book should be on the shelf of everyone who is dealing with, or may have to deal with, a loved one who is dying."

Jean Layland, Baytext Communications

INTRODUCTION

The idea for this book first began to develop in 1997. My mother's breast cancer had returned, spreading to her lungs and liver. She was given a matter of months to live.

As our family tried to grapple with the heartbreaking news, I realized that I had absolutely no idea what to do. My mother was in pain and growing weaker by the day. My brain was no longer functioning – muddled by the grief and anguish of the situation. I wanted someone to tell me what to do, to help me focus on the most important things in the time that remained.

I went to the library and to local bookstores looking for a guide – a book that would help me organize my thoughts and give support and comfort to my mother. I found books about the process of grieving and loss, about death and dying, but nothing that walked me through the practical things that I needed to do for my mother, for my family and for me before she died.

Afterwards, a whole new set of tasks needed to be taken care of. I had never planned a funeral before, and had no idea how gut-wrenching the process could be. Banks and credit card companies needed to be contacted. My brother and I had to go through her personal belongings. The affairs of her estate needed to be managed, all of these tasks – needing to be done – in the midst of overwhelming pain, anger and depression.

This book is a response to the void I experienced when my mother died. It provides the framework I so desperately wished someone had given me. The book is divided into two parts. Part I focuses on the most important things in the time that remains after a loved one has been diagnosed with a life-threatening illness. It includes advice on a wide range of topics such as dealing with healthcare professionals, identifying sources of financial assistance, clarifying your loved one's final wishes and directives, and taking the time to preserve memories.

Part II of the book addresses what happens after your loved one dies. It walks you through the decisions and tasks that need to be addressed including caring for the body, planning a funeral, dealing with grief and executing a will.

At the back of the book, you'll find forms that can be copied to help you manage the practical things that need to be taken care of, such as creating a contact list of healthcare professionals, tracking medications, advance planning of arrangements after death and writing an obituary. This book is not intended to replace advice from doctors, lawyers, accountants or other professionals. It simply offers practical suggestions, checklists and forms to help you think through tasks and take care of the most important things.

Some of the topics may be extremely difficult to talk about. However, working through important questions and understanding the final wishes of your loved one can help with the decisions and arrangements to be made in the time that remains, and provide peace of mind for you and for them.

While the book has been written from a North American perspective, the information and practical suggestions may be helpful to people from a variety of places, faiths and cultures.

Each person and each circumstance is unique. Some of the chapters may not be relevant to your situation. Choose the topics and issues that best meet your needs.

It is my hope that this book will help guide both family and friends as you seek to care for your loved one in the time that remains and honour their wishes after death.

Jeanne M. Sedun

TABLE OF CONTENTS

Part One
The Time That Remains

Focusing on the Most Important Things

CHAPTER 1

Where to Begin

Time is the most valuable thing a man can spend.

Laertius Diogenes

A loved one has been diagnosed with a terminal illness. They – and you – must face the prospect of their imminent death. What do you do now?

Part I of this book is intended to help you and your loved one focus on the most important things in the time that remains. It walks you through some of the practical things that you'll need to think about, and provides some suggestions on how to cope.

WHAT YOU MAY BE FEELING

Before focusing your attention on the things that need to be done, take a moment to reflect on what you're feeling. It can be extremely difficult to come to terms with the fact that someone you love has been diagnosed with a life-threatening illness. One of the common reactions to events like this is anticipatory grief – intense sorrow knowing that someone you love is dying.

Here are some of the things you may be feeling:

- shock and numbness;
- anxiety and fear about death, pain and suffering, and what life will be like without them;
- anger and sadness about why this is happening;
- denial and an unwillingness to believe that the diagnosis is accurate;
- an inability to cope with daily activities, and a feeling of being overwhelmed; and
- despair and hopelessness.

A terminal illness has a physical and emotional impact on family and friends as well. Understanding and acknowledging your feelings is an important part of caring for your loved one. Allowing others to help you in ways that are meaningful for you is also important, since taking care of yourself will help you be able to support and care for your loved one.

Some practical ways that you can take care of yourself include:

- making time for regular exercise to help your body be strong and to relieve stress;
- maintaining a good diet and stocking up on healthy snacks such as fruit and protein bars, since you may not always be able to eat at regular times;
- doing things that sooth you, like playing an instrument, talking with a friend, having a massage or meditating;
- keeping up with your dental and medical appointments;
- going for counselling or joining a support group; and,
- asking family and friends for help with shopping, meals and household chores.

WHAT YOUR LOVED ONE MAY BE FEELING

Expressing emotions and feelings can be difficult – especially in times of crisis. You and your loved one may be experiencing a whole range of constantly changing emotions – fear, anxiety and anger. It is sometimes easier to talk about almost anything except the fact that someone you love is dying.

Dying is a new experience to which each person reacts differently. It's difficult to know what to say. Some people facing life-threatening illnesses are comfortable talking about their own feelings and allowing others to share theirs openly. Other people choose to keep their thoughts and feelings to themselves. Listening – to whatever your loved one chooses to talk about – is one of the key ways you can support them.

FIVE STAGES OF DYING

Five stages of dying were identified by Dr. Elisabeth Kübler-Ross, who spent years working with terminally ill children, AIDS patients and the elderly. These stages describe the behaviour and thinking of a person who is dying: denial and isolation, anger, bargaining, depression, and acceptance.

- **Denial and isolation** - In the first stage of dying, a person denies that death is going to take place. This is a common reaction to a diagnosis of a terminal illness. a
- **Anger** - Denial then gives way to anger and resentment, when a person recognizes that they are in fact dying. At this point, some people take their anger out on medical staff, family members or friends.
- **Bargaining** - The third stage involves bargaining where a person hopes that death can somehow be postponed or delayed by leading a reformed life or making better choices.
- **Depression** - As the person comes to accept the certainty of death, depression may set in. Behaviours may include frequent crying and withdrawal as the person contemplates their impending death.

- **Acceptance** - In the fifth stage of dying, the person learns to accept their fate, and develops a sense of peace.

You may realize that your loved one is still wrestling with issues such as denial or anger. People don't necessarily work through all five stages, or go through them in the order they have been described above. The stages model can be helpful in making some sense of the thoughts and emotions that your loved one may be experiencing.

There are other models that go beyond the stages and emotions described by Kübler-Ross. A person's personality and experiences impact their approach to death and dying. It is important to remember that each person experiences their death journey in their own way.

Reflecting on one's life – events, successes and failures, and relationships – is a process that often happens spontaneously once a person is diagnosed with a terminal illness. Working through complicated and overwhelming feelings is part of the dying process. Your loved one may find it helpful to sort through their life's experiences and make sense of their thoughts and feelings by considering a series of emotional and psychological questions developed by Dr. David Kuhl in his book entitled *Facing Death, Embracing Life*. The questions include a focus on understanding oneself, the yearning to belong and the need to be loved – particularly at the end of life.

Communicating with a Loved One Who is Dying

CARE AND COMFORT	CONSIDERATION
Touch	Holding a hand or offering an embrace can create a strong sense of connection with others. It can counteract the sense of isolation or aloneness that your loved one may be feeling.
Physical presence	Sitting with your loved one, even if they are silent, can give a sense of comfort and support.
Humour	Reminiscing about a humorous event or watching a favorite funny movie can lift a person's mood and help your loved one focus on something other than their pain or discomfort.
Active listening	Being an active listener may help your loved one to talk about their fears and concerns.
Friendship	Providing help with letter-writing, phone calls and visits can help your loved one stay in touch with friends.

CARE AND COMFORT	CONSIDERATION
Favourite activities	Arranging for your loved one to experience their favourite activities such as music, movies or books on tape can help them find enjoyment.
Cards / notes	Sending cards of encouragement and support can be an opportunity to show appreciation for the person and to express the impact the person has had on the lives of others.

It is important to maintain open communication with a person who is dying, including helping your loved one and significant others to understand that the person is in fact dying. Being open and honest allows the dying person to end their life in a way that respects their personal ideas and values. It gives them the opportunity to complete a cherished project, get their affairs in order, make arrangements for survivors, or participate in decisions about arrangements after death. It also provides an opportunity to reflect on life and to express emotions that may have gone unspoken.

Beyond open communication, there are some simple things that family and friends can do to provide care and comfort to your loved one at the end of life.

TALKING WITH CHILDREN ABOUT DEATH AND DYING

Children are impacted as well when someone is diagnosed with a life-threatening illness. They can often sense that something is wrong. Reactions may vary depending on age, experiences and personality.

Death is a natural part of life – one that children experience from a young age when they see dead birds or insects, or have to bury to a family pet. By talking with children about death and dying, you can give them the freedom to ask questions and discuss their feelings openly. Answers to their questions should be brief and at a level that they can understand.

Giving a child meaningful opportunities to care for a loved one or to say goodbye can help them understand and accept death. Consider including them in activities or visits with your loved one. There are also some excellent resources available to help you talk with children about death and dying (see *Appendix 2: Reading List – Talking with Children about Death and Dying*).

SUPPORT FROM FRIENDS AND FAMILY

Caring for a terminally ill loved one can be emotionally and physically exhausting. Unfortunately, many caregivers are often hesitant to ask for assistance from friends and family. Don't be afraid to ask for help.

Here are some practical suggestions for friends and family about how they can provide assistance.

- **Groceries** – Offer to pick up groceries and help put them away.
- **Meals** – Drop off prepared meals that can quickly be reheated.
- **Childcare** – Arrange a fun outing for any children in the home.
- **Vehicle maintenance** – Take care of basic vehicle maintenance such as arranging for an oil change or car wash.
- **House maintenance** – Offer to rake leaves, clean gutters or take care of flower beds.
- **Pampering** – Give a gift certificate for a massage or manicure to the caregiver so they can take a much-needed break. Offer to care for the terminally-ill person while the caregiver is gone.

It's a good idea to arrange for someone to coordinate any offers of assistance. This will allow for the coordination of meal deliveries, streamline the sharing of updates on the person's health and prevent the phone from ringing endlessly.

CHAPTER 2

Medical Care

Everything that happens to us leaves some trace behind; everything contributes imperceptibly to make us what we are.

Johann Wolfgang von Goethe

It can feel overwhelming dealing with the care of someone who is seriously ill or dying. The following section will help you understand the areas of expertise of some of the medical specialists you may be encountering. You'll also find some advice on talking with medical staff, along with suggestions for managing medical appointments and administering medications.

HEALTHCARE PROFESSIONALS

It's important to talk with the health professionals involved. Patients and their loved ones need to be well informed in order to make the best decisions possible under the circumstances.

Some of the healthcare professionals you will likely encounter include:

General practitioner

A general practitioner or family doctor is often the first point of contact for non-emergency medical problems. In many cases, it's the family doctor who initially investigates an abnormality or illness, orders preliminary tests, and provides a referral to one or more medical specialists.

Specialist

A specialist is a doctor who has completed medical school and then gone on to take additional training in a specific field. *Appendix 1* provides a listing of some of the more common types of medical specialists along with a brief description of their area of expertise.

Home care nurse

A home care nurse provides care to patients in their home, working under the direction of a doctor. Services may range from homemaking services such as cooking and cleaning, to personal and medical care.

Patient navigator

Patient navigators are specially trained healthcare providers like registered nurses or social workers who help patients with access to care and services. They provide patients with a single point of contact for questions, and work one-on-one with patients including assessing needs, coordinating tests and liaising with doctors to prevent patients from falling through the cracks.

COMMUNICATING EFFECTIVELY WITH MEDICAL STAFF

Here are some suggestions to ensure effective communication with medical staff:

- Think about questions and concerns in advance. What kind of information do you want from the doctors or nurses (e.g., treatment options, available support services)? Is there some relevant information about your loved one's condition or situation that you need to communicate? Consider writing down your thoughts to get the most out of your discussions with the health professionals.
- Attend medical appointments with your loved one, if they will allow you to. These appointments can be disheartening, particularly if the diagnosis is not good. Being available to drive and attend these appointments can be an important source of support and comfort for your loved one.
- Take notes. It can be difficult to absorb everything that's said during interactions with health professionals, particularly when someone is seriously ill or dying. Writing down the interactions and comments will help you remember what was said, and can be useful when talking with other family members or friends about the diagnosis and recommended course of treatment.

Some doctors will allow you to tape their advice, especially when they're discussing complex options. Always ask before recording the interaction.

- Be persistent. Keep asking questions if you don't feel that the health professionals are being completely up front with you, or if there is something you don't understand.
- Request copies of key medical documents. Many healthcare providers allow patients to request copies of surgical, pathology or lab reports.
- Be aware of your feelings. Emotions can be very strong when someone you love is seriously ill. Directing anger or frustration at medical staff won't help the situation. However, it is important to acknowledge your feelings and to find constructive ways to care for your physical and emotional health and well-being (see *Chapter 9: Grief and Grieving*)

Form 1: Discussions with Healthcare Professionals provides one option for tracking this information. A completed sample is shown below.

Form 1: Discussions with Healthcare Professionals

DATE	DOCTOR	COMMENTS	NEXT STEPS
February 3	Dr. Smith (family doctor)	Blood tests to be completed this week.	Dr. Smith will review blood test results and then consider changes to medication, if required.
February 10	Dr. Franklin (radiologist)	Need to increase the frequency of radiation treatments.	Dr. Franklin's office will call with a revised radiation treatment schedule.
February 11	Dr. Jones (oncologist)	6-week chemotherapy treatment has been unsuccessful.	Consider different chemotherapy treatment starting next week. OK to take a day or two to think about it. Need to phone Dr. Jones office if agree to proceed with new treatment.

Make sure you have the contact information for each health professional involved in the care of your loved one. It is helpful to clarify each person's role in the treatment, and under what circumstances you should contact them, e.g., pain management. **Form 2: Medical Specialists Contact List** provides a template for tracking this information. A completed sample is shown on the following page. Another option is to get a business card from each healthcare professional, and keep the cards in an organizer so that the contact information is always readily available.

Form 2: Medical Specialists Contact List

SPECIALIST	FUNCTION	ADDRESS	TEL / FAX
John Smith	Family doctor – manages general health issues; makes referrals to medical specialists; monitors blood test results.	#3 – 114 Cortez Road	Tel: 356-4322 Fax: 356-4387
Barbara Jones	Oncologist – works with the cancer clinic; responsible for surgery and chemotherapy treatments.	Cancer Clinic #306 764 Cranberry Lane	Tel: 985-4824 Fax: 985-4825
Jody Franklin	Radiologist – oversees radiation treatments at the cancer clinic.	Cancer Clinic #507 764 Cranberry Lane	Tel: 985-4857 Fax: 985-4858

TRACKING MEDICAL INFORMATION AND APPOINTMENTS

You will need to keep track of many unfamiliar things regarding the health of your loved one. It's helpful to keep the forms and all medical information in a central binder, with tabs for appointments, medications, reports, specialist opinions, correspondence, lab results, etc. This will provide a central place where all of the information is readily accessible, helping to ensure that nothing falls through the cracks. When emotions run high, it's easy to misinterpret or forget important information. Careful record keeping will make things much easier for you and your loved one.

Keeping track of appointments can become challenging when you're dealing with a variety of medical specialists. Consider purchasing a wallet-sized planner or a small calendar that will fit into a purse or coat pocket so that all of the relevant appointments are tracked in one place. It's helpful to take the calendar with you to each appointment to avoid scheduling conflicts. If you've chosen to use a central binder, you may wish to hole-punch the planner or calendar and keep it in the binder or file it in a folder insert designed to store miscellaneous documents at the back of the binder.

ADMINISTERING MEDICATION

It's important to manage medications properly in order to maximize their benefits for your loved one. Here are a few things to keep in mind when helping with medications:

- **Store the medications properly**. Watch for special storage instructions, such as a requirement to keep the medicine refrigerated. Ensure that medicine is kept out of the reach of children.
- **Administer the correct medicine**. Check the label each time a medication is given to make sure that it is the prescribed medicine and that the correct amount is being given. This is especially important when dealing with multiple medications in containers that look similar.
- **Take note of any special instructions**. Some medications have special instructions such as a requirement to take with food or shake before administering. This can impact the effectiveness of the medication.
- **Avoid drug interactions**. Make sure that the doctors are aware of all medications and/or herbal remedies being given in order to avoid negative drug interactions. It's also a good idea to consult with the pharmacist who can print out a list of the medications and review them with you. **Be aware of side effects**. Ask about any potential side effects when getting a prescription filled, so you are aware of what to watch out for.
- **Watch for expiry dates**. Medications have expiry dates indicating when the drug is too old to use. If a medication is outdated, it may be less effective or even harmful.
- **Use a medication dispenser**. A pill dispenser can help organize medications by day of the week and by time of day (e.g., morning, afternoon or evening). This is particularly helpful if your loved one is taking a variety of medications.
- **Track medication supplies**. It might take a few days to get a prescription refilled. Keeping track of medication stocks will ensure that a new supply can be ordered before the current supply runs out.
- **Keep a medication schedule**. Creating a medication schedule can help you remember the timing for each medication along with the dosage, and can serve as a reminder for any special instructions. **Form 3: Medication Schedule** provides a template for tracking this information. A completed sample is shown on the following page.

Form 3: Medication Schedule

MEDICATION	DOSAGE	DIRECTIONS	PURPOSE	12 AM	2 AM	4 AM	6 AM	8 AM	10 AM	12 PM	2 PM	4 PM	6 PM	8 PM	10 PM
Tamoxifen	1 - 10mg tablet	Take orally twice a day with food or on an empty stomach with a glass of water or juice.	Cancer-fighting agent					✓						✓	
Aspirin	2 - 400mg tablets	Take orally every 4-6 hours as needed, to a maximum of 4,000mg per day.	Pain management					✓			✓			✓	
Gravol	1 - 100 mg caplet	Take orally every 8 hours as needed to a maximum of 400 mg in 24 hours.	Nausea					✓						✓	

MONITORING HEALTH CHANGES

Careful monitoring of any unusual reactions or changes in the condition of your loved one provides valuable information when meeting with medical staff, and can assist doctors in tailoring medication. Things to watch for include:

- Sensitivities or negative reactions to medication, such as nausea, swelling, and skin rashes;
- Symptoms including headaches, weight loss, weight gain, pain while swallowing, change in bowel movements, limb weakness or memory problems; and,
- Changes in diet, appetite, stress or mood.

Form 4: Monitoring Health Changes provides one option for tracking this information. A completed sample is shown below.

Form 4: Monitoring Health Changes

DATE	TIME	SYMPTOM / REACTION	CIRCUMSTANCE
September 6	8:30am	Nausea	Felt ill after taking morning dose of Tamoxifen at 8am
September 6	3:30pm	Headache	Developed a nasty headache while reading; took aspirin
September 8	2:00am	Night sweats	Woke up at 2am sweating and very hot; couldn't sleep

MEDICAL CARE OPTIONS

There may come a time when your loved one requires assistance managing their personal and medical care. There are several options to consider.

Home care nursing program

In some cases, home support is available to assist with health services and daily activities so patients can stay in their homes as long as possible.

Some of the services that may be available include:

- Home support (meals, light housekeeping, laundry);
- Personal care assistance (transferring to/from a wheelchair, bathing);
- Healthcare (counselling, nursing care); and,
- Medication, supplies and equipment.

Home care nursing programs generally require an assessment of existing supports and community services. Ask your family doctor or regional health authority for information on home care nursing programs in your area.

Assisted living suites

Some communities offer assisted living suites for people who are able to live in a semi-independent environment. Assisted living combines housing, meals, housekeeping and any personal services that may be needed, such as bathing and dressing, laundry, bill payment or medication management. Rooms are generally unfurnished, and usually feature bathrooms with safety bars, a 24/7 emergency response system, and medical staff on duty 24 hours a day in case of emergency.

Long-term care home

When a person can no longer remain safely at home, even with home care or assisted living services, placement in a long-term personal care home may be an option. Long-term care homes are designed for people who require the availability of 24-hour nursing care and supervision. Fees vary depending on the type of accommodation selected, e.g., private, semi-private or ward. Subsidies may be available for people with lower incomes. Check with your local health authority for information on admission to government-subsidized nursing homes.

If there are a number of personal care home facilities in your community, consider visiting several of them before deciding where your loved one will be placed. Be aware that many personal care homes have waiting lists, so placement is sometimes delayed.

Hospice

A hospice is a special healthcare facility that looks after people who need care at the end stage of a terminal illness. The focus of care is on comfort and improving the quality of life. Hospice rooms are often decorated to create a more welcoming environment than a hospital room, but are not intended for longer-term stays.

Admission to a hospice facility is often arranged through home and community care nurses, or through a doctor or nurse in a palliative care program – a program focused on helping relieve the symptoms and side effects of disease, especially for people diagnosed with terminal illnesses. People admitted to a hospice are not seeking medical help to prolong their lives, and are generally expected to live less than 3 weeks. Many insurance companies and provincial or state funded medical care programs cover the basic costs of hospice care.

CHAPTER 3

Financial Assistance

If we are facing in the right direction, all we have to do is keep on walking.

Zen Proverb

A serious illness can have a devastating effect on personal finances. The loss of income, plus expenses for medications and travel associated with medical treatments, can place a severe strain on the financial and emotional well-being of your loved one. There are a couple of options you may wish to explore in order to help them cope with the financial strain.

DISABILITY INSURANCE

Check to see if your loved one has disability insurance. This type of insurance is sometimes included as part of an employee benefits plan. Some disability insurance policies only cover disability resulting from an accident, whereas other policies cover disability from a prolonged illness. Check with your loved one's employer or the insurance company providing the group insurance for information on any coverage that may be available.

COMPASSIONATE CARE PROGRAMS

Some companies and/or jurisdictions offer a compassionate care benefit program for people caring for a family member who is terminally ill and at risk of dying. In many cases, the program provides funding to allow a person to take a temporary leave from work to provide care or support to an immediate family member. Medical documentation is usually required, confirming that your loved one is gravely ill with a significant risk of dying. The medical certificate may also need to indicate that they require assistance from one or more family members.

Contact your employer or your local employment office to determine whether you might be eligible for funding to take time off work to care for your loved one.

DISABILITY BENEFITS PROGRAMS

Many jurisdictions offer disability benefits programs with accelerated review and approval procedures for terminally ill patients. For example, the Canada Pension Plan has a disability component that provides a monthly payment to eligible contributors who cannot work because of a severe and prolonged disability that may result in death. Applicants with a terminal illness have their disability applications reviewed within 48 hours upon receipt of their application.

In the United States, the Social Security Disability Insurance Program provides disability benefits in the form of monthly payments for eligible terminally ill individuals. Once again, there is an expedited process for processing terminally ill cases. Contact your local federal office to explore whether your loved one is eligible for disability benefits. Other countries, such as the United Kingdom, have similar programs.

PALLIATIVE CARE BENEFIT PROGRAMS

Some jurisdictions have special programs that cover the cost of medications for terminally ill people registered in palliative care programs. The focus of care in this type of program is on comfort rather than curing or treating the illness. Palliative care addresses the physical symptoms and side effects of disease, as well as emotional, social and spiritual suffering in order to achieve the best possible quality of life. By covering the cost of eligible drugs, these programs remove a major financial burden for the patient and their family. The criteria for eligibility vary by jurisdiction, although it is often a requirement that the application form be completed by a physician. Your loved one's doctor should be able to provide information on the availability of any palliative care benefit programs in your area. Information on palliative care organizations is included in *Appendix 4* and *Appendix 5*.

OTHER FUNDING SOURCES

In some instances, organizations such as the local cancer agency have programs available to assist with treatment-related travel and accommodation expenses or the cost of medications. This often involves a confidential needs assessment, requiring information on household income, in order to assess the patient's eligibility for a financial subsidy. Another potential source of income might be the investment component of a whole life insurance plan (refer to the section on Life Insurance Policies). Your family doctor or medical specialist may be able to provide additional information on other sources of funding that might be available.

CHAPTER 4

Important Documents and Information

The whole of life is but a moment of time. It is our duty, therefore to use it, not to misuse it.

Plutarch

Working with your loved one to locate and organize important documents and information in the time that remains can make it easier for friends and family to carry out their wishes after death. Having to search through boxes, files and correspondence to locate key documents after death can create unnecessary tension and heartache in the midst of grief and sadness.

Arranging the affairs of your loved one can be so much easier if you have the opportunity to talk with them – to work through this process with them. They may not be prepared to talk about their affairs, or to provide information on their financial situation. Be sensitive to their willingness to consider the following items.

KEY CONTACTS

It's helpful to create a master list of the key contacts in your loved one's life.

The list should include people who are important to them, like close friends and work colleagues, as well as key advisors such as a lawyer or accountant. This information will help you manage their affairs in the time that remains and after death. Consider including the following people:

- Family
- Friends
- Work colleagues
- Minister or spiritual advisor
- Executor
- Person with power of attorney for health/finances
- Accountant
- Lawyer
- Banker
- Insurance agent
- Investment advisor

Form 5: Key Contacts provides a template for gathering this information. A sample is shown below.

Form 5: Listing of Key Contacts

NAME	RELATIONSHIP	TELEPHONE	EMAIL
Geoffrey Arnauld	Brother	204-382-1999	Garnauld@mail.com
Katie Acheson	Best friend	312-487-1321	ka@friend.com
Jordan Hinds	Lawyer Hinds and Blaney Law Associates	250-387-7532	Jhinds@legal.com
Reverend John Willis	Minister Fairwinds United Church	250-987-6543	revwillis@church.com

Identification papers

It's important to keep your loved one's identification papers safe and secure before and after death to prevent situations such as identity theft. These papers include their driver's licence, birth certificate and marriage certificate, as well as passport and citizenship documents. Ideally, find out where these documents are kept and work with your loved one to ensure they are in a safe place. This is particularly important if your loved one is in a public care setting such as a hospital or nursing home, where theft is an unfortunate reality.

FINANCIAL INFORMATION

Understanding your loved one's financial situation – what they own (assets) and what they owe (liabilities) – is an important step in helping them manage their finances and plan for what happens to their assets after death.

Bank account information

It's not uncommon for people to have several bank accounts with different banking institutions. Gathering basic information such as the name and contact information for each financial institution, along with information about the account type, number and ownership can help with the management of your loved one's affairs.

Joint ownership of bank accounts can make it easier to access funds both before and after death. However, it's important to ensure the trustworthiness of anyone being given joint account ownership to ensure that they have the best interests of your loved one at heart.

Form 6: Bank Account Information provides a template for gathering this information. A completed sample is shown below.

Form 6: Bank Account Information

FINANCIAL INSTITUTION	Marina Credit Union	
ADDRESS	123 Strawberry Vale, Mittlenatch, BC V7M 7Y7	
TEL / FAX / EMAIL	Tel: 386-7954; Fax: 386-7955; Email: customer@marinacu.com	
ACCOUNT TYPE	ACCOUNT NUMBER	OWNERSHIP
Chequing	987654	Joint with daughter Susan
Savings	876543	Individual

Insurance policies

Insurance policies can provide for the financial needs of surviving loved ones, such as money for education or funds to pay off a mortgage. In some cases, an insurance policy can also provide a source of funding here and now.

Types of life insurance

Life insurance is a legal contract between a policy owner and an insurance company that guarantees a specific sum of money be paid to a person (called a designated beneficiary) upon the death of the insured. There are two basic types of life insurance – term insurance and whole life insurance.

Term insurance provides temporary insurance protection and pays a predetermined amount if the insured dies during a specified period of time. Monthly insurance payments, called premiums, may have been set up to be paid automatically from your loved one's bank account. This type of insurance is sometimes also included as part of an employee benefits plan, with monthly premiums being paid directly by the employer.

Whole life insurance provides permanent coverage that remains in effect for the entire life of the insured. The premiums cover the insurance risk along with a savings or investment component, which increases in value over time. Funds can be borrowed from the savings portion of the insurance if your loved one is experiencing financial difficulties due to their illness.

Universal life insurance is a variation on whole life insurance. It provides permanent coverage, but with more flexible premiums and benefits. The policy holder is able to shift money between the insurance and the savings component of the policy.

If your loved one purchased a whole life insurance policy some time ago, it's possible that the policy premiums have been paid in full and monthly premiums are no longer being deducted from their account. It is therefore quite important that you talk with your loved one to identify any life insurance policies that may exist – including policies purchased some time ago or policies that are included as part of an employee benefits package.

Your loved one may wish to review the beneficiary information for their life insurance plans, and consider specifying named beneficiaries (i.e., specific individuals or entities such as a charity) that will receive the sum specified in the policy. This will ensure that funds can be paid directly to the beneficiaries without waiting for the estate to be settled. It also prevents the funds from becoming part of the estate and being subject to probate fees or the claims of creditors. Your loved one may wish to discuss any changes to their life insurance coverage, including designating beneficiaries, with an experienced life insurance agent.

Form 7: Life Insurance Policies provides a template for gathering this information. A completed sample is shown below.

Form 7: Life Insurance Policy Information

INSURANCE COMPANY	*Sunshine Life Insurance Company*
TYPE OF INSURANCE (Term, Whole Life, Universal)	*Whole life*
POLICY VALUE	*$125,000; $50,000 cash value available if need to borrow funds now to cover living expenses*
POLICY NUMBER	*543210-003*
BENEFICIARY	*No named beneficiary*
POLICY LOCATION	*Life insurance file in basement filing cabinet*
INSURANCE AGENT	*Jack Simpson*
TEL / FAX / EMAIL	*Tel: 475-9898; Fax: 475-9900; Email: info@SunshineInsurance.com*

Borrowing from a life insurance policy

It may be possible to borrow from an existing whole life insurance policy if the policy has built up a cash value. The advantage of borrowing against the cash value of a policy is that you do not have to repay the loan during your lifetime. The disadvantage is that a loan against a policy decreases the death benefit available if the loan is not repaid in full before the insured dies. The insurance company may also charge interest on the money borrowed.

Life insurance for the terminally ill

The option of purchasing traditional life insurance is generally not available for a person diagnosed with a terminal illness. However, some companies offer a graded benefit life insurance policy for the terminally ill. With this type of policy, a percentage of the death benefit becomes available each year. This means that if the insured dies during the first two years the policy is in effect, the amount paid out will be less than the full amount. Policies for a terminally ill person are more expensive than policies for a healthy person of the same age, since the policyholder presents greater risk to the insurance company. The death benefit available is also limited.

Other types of insurance

Check whether existing credit cards and loans carry credit life insurance, which is used to pay off these debts in the event of death.

Investments

Gathering and organizing basic information on your loved one's investments can make it easier to fulfill your loved one's wishes for distributing their assets. This information includes things like the names of the investment firms, the types of accounts and account ownership (e.g., individual or joint). Investments that you'll want to take note of include retirement and education savings plans, annuities, stocks and bonds.

Form 8: Investment Account Information provides a template for gathering this information. A completed sample is shown below.

Form 8: Investment Account Information

INVESTMENT FIRM	Mountainview Bank	
INVESTMENT ADVISOR	Sidney Pettigrew	
ADDRESS	#3 - 487 Frame Road, Seagull Harbour	
TEL / FAX / EMAIL	Tel: 323-4875; Fax: 323-4876; Email: customer@mountainviewbank.com	
ACCOUNT TYPE	ACCOUNT NUMBER	OWNERSHIP
Registered Retirement Savings Plan	6529876	Individual
Registered Education Savings Plan	47593-002	Beneficiary: Daughter Guinevere

INVESTMENT FIRM	Bull's-eye Investments	
INVESTMENT ADVISOR	Dorothy Langton	
ADDRESS	75 Misty Lane, Franklin Bay	
TEL / FAX / EMAIL	Tel: 444-3795; Fax: 444-3800; Email: mail@bullseye.net	
ACCOUNT TYPE	ACCOUNT NUMBER	OWNERSHIP
Savings bonds	123-123456	Single ownership
Mutual funds	ABC789	Co-owned with partner

Information on other investments such as savings bonds, share certificates, pensions plans and annuities can be tracked using **Form 9: Other Investments**. A completed sample is shown below.

Form 9: Other Investments

COMPANY	Federal government	
CONTACT	Nick Grundfeld	
TEL / FAX / EMAIL	Tel: 1-800-987-6543; info available on web at federalgovernmentbonds.com	
DESCRIPTION	POLICY / PLAN #	DOCUMENT LOCATION
Savings bonds	FG2014-10	Filing cabinet in den

COMPANY	Green Day Pension Corporation	
CONTACT	Cynthia Bradshaw	
TEL / FAX / EMAIL	Tel: 1-800-992-6933; Email: contact@greenday.ca	
DESCRIPTION	POLICY / PLAN #	DOCUMENT LOCATION
Company pension plan - Smith & Smith Machinery	41799	Pension plan documents in den filing cabinet

Other Assets

There are other assets that should also be taken into consideration when working through the financial affairs of your loved one, such as vehicles, art, antiques, furniture, jewellery and coin collections. These assets are often specifically identified in a will if they are of significant value, along with a named beneficiary for specific items such as a cherished ring or a family heirloom. Be specific about the description of the item in order to avoid any potential confusion or conflicts about the distribution of your loved one's assets.

Form 10: Valuable Personal Assets provides a template for listing this information. A completed sample is shown in below.

Form 10: Valuable Personal Assets

ITEM DESCRIPTION	LOCATION	BENEFICIARY
Grandma Elsie's 18" black pearl necklace with silver clasp	Safe deposit box – Mountainview Bank	Daughter Guinevere
14' aluminum boat with storage cover, 3hp motor, trailer and 4 fishing rods	Covered storage shed in backyard	Son Stanley
Landscape painting by Cynthia MacDougall (my favourite painting)	Hanging in front entrance hallway	Katrina Atkins (family friend)

REAL ESTATE

Real estate holdings, if any, should also be identified. This includes basic information on your loved one's principal residence, along with any vacation or investment properties. In addition to sole ownership, there are various other forms of property ownership to consider.

Joint tenancy

In joint tenancy, a piece of property is owned by one or more people, with each person having an equal entitlement to the property. If the property is owned by several people and any one person dies, the remaining owners or joint tenants automatically and equally take over that person's interest in the property. This is also known as the "rule of survivorship" since the property does not go to the heirs of a deceased person. Joint tenancy is one means of passing property along after death without having to go through probate.

Tenants in common

If one tenant or co-owner dies, their share of the property goes to their estate and beneficiaries. There is no rule of survivorship. Tenants in common is one way of passing along shares or portions of ownership in a family cabin that in turn could be bequeathed to subsequent generations.

Condominium ownership

Ownership of properties like condominiums, lofts and townhouses gives title or ownership of an individual unit within a building, along with an interest in the condominium corporation that owns the common elements of the building or community. The owner has responsibility for maintaining their unit, and is required to pay a monthly fee to the condominium corporation as their share of the expenses to maintain the common elements.

Life interest

This type of ownership gives a person the right to live in, occupy or use a piece of property for as long as they live. Upon death, they lose all rights to the property.

Form 11: Real Estate Assets provides a template for identifying this information. A completed sample is shown below.

Form 11: Real Estate Assets

TYPE OF PROPERTY	Principal residence
ADDRESS	7642 Maple Street, Lanson Island
OWNER(S)	Nathan Herd and Helga Clement
FORM OF OWNERSHIP	Joint tenancy
DEED LOCATION	Safe deposit box, Mountainview Bank
MORTGAGE COMPANY	Reliable Mortgage Financial Corporation
MORTGAGE REF. #	3100111
TEL / FAX / EMAIL	Tel: 1-800-285-5432; Email: contact@reliablemortgage.net
CONTACT	Graham Dickens

Liabilities

Understanding the financial liabilities or debts of your loved one becomes particularly important if you are responsible for managing their financial affairs during their illness. This might include paying household bills such as hydro and telephone service, as well as payments for a mortgage, loan or credit cards. Keeping monthly payments up to date will ensure that services are not cut off, creating additional and unnecessary stress. There may be arrangements to pay some of the bills through an automatic deduction. Knowing about these arrangements will help you better monitor your loved one's financial position.

Form 12: Bills to be Paid provides a template for listing and tracking your loved one's bills. A completed sample is shown below.

Form 12: Bills to be Paid

DESCRIPTION	ACCOUNT #	CONTACT INFO	AMOUNT	DUE DATE
Reliable Mortgage Financial Corporation (mortgage on house)	3100111	Graham Dickens Tel: 285-5432	$850	1st and 15th of each month
Autumn Telephone Company (telephone and long distance)	4329876	1-888-987-6543	$35	15th
Island Hydro (heat and electricity)	9998876	1-800-123-4567 Monthly payment plan	$199	28th

ESTATE PLANNING

Now that you and your loved one have a basic understanding of their financial situation, including what they own and what they owe, you will be able to help them plan for the transfer of their assets upon death. Estate planning allows a person to specify what they want to happen to their assets when they die, and can also help manage the tax consequences of the asset transfers. Consider seeking advice from an estate attorney and a financial professional with expertise in estate planning.

An estate is made up of the assets or items a person owns at death as well as the personal debts or liabilities owed. The first step in estate planning is figuring out a person's net worth. The financial information referenced earlier in this chapter will help you and your loved one calculate their net worth by subtracting the total liabilities or money owed from the total of all of their assets.

The following forms will help when you work with your loved one to figure out their financial situation:

Form 13: Assets and Liabilities Checklist; and, **Form 14: Calculating Net Worth**.

CHAPTER 5

Final Wishes and Advance Directives

There is only one thing that remains to us, that cannot be taken away: to act with courage and dignity and to stick to the ideals that have given meaning to life.

Jawaharlal Nehru

It can be very difficult to bring up the subject of getting your loved one's affairs in order. It may feel as though dealing with financial and legal matters is an admission that death is drawing near. Your loved one may be reluctant to talk about such matters. You yourself may feel hesitant to bring up the subject. However, working through some key questions and understanding the final wishes of your loved one can help with the decisions and arrangements to be made in the time that remains, and provide peace of mind for both you and your loved one.

A WILL

A will is one of the key documents for putting a person's affairs in order. It is a legal document that specifies how to distribute a person's assets upon death. It allows for the selection of an executor to administer the estate. This is the person responsible for carrying out the wishes of your loved one after they die. A will can help avoid confusion and reduce family conflict over the distribution of assets. The terms *will* and *testament* are sometimes used interchangeably.

The job of an executor can be very challenging depending on family dynamics and the complexity of the estate. Some people choose a family member or friend as the executor, while others prefer to appoint a lawyer or accountant – particularly if there may be conflicts over what is to be inherited and by whom. Without a will, the court will select an estate administrator. It is also likely that there will be delays in the distribution of the estate, along with higher administration costs.

Many people choose to have a will drawn up by a lawyer, particularly if their estate is large. Here are some things to consider when drawing up or revising a will:

- Are there other wills in existence that need to be revoked?
- Are there certain gifts, personal or household effects (e.g., jewellery), property, etc. that are to be given to a specified beneficiary or charity?
- Has a guardian been appointed for children who are minors, in the event that your loved one and their spouse die at the same time?
- Has an executor been appointed, and is there a description of their role and responsibilities?
- Does the executor have the freedom to use their discretion in managing the estate assets? Is the executor is to be released from any loss that might happen as a result of estate management decisions?

Once a will has been drawn up, it's important to keep it in a place that is easily accessible. Consider providing copies of the will to the executor and beneficiaries. If the will is in a safe-deposit box, a court order may be needed to release the contents, unless the box is jointly held.

Some people choose to talk with the executor or discuss the provisions of the will with the beneficiaries in order to avoid conflict or misunderstandings. Think about what would best fit with the wishes and interests of your loved one.

POWER OF ATTORNEY

A power of attorney is a legal document that authorizes someone else to carry out decisions and manage financial and most legal decisions on behalf of your loved one. This authorization may include access to bank accounts, paying bills and making financial decisions, but does not include medical or healthcare decisions. A power of attorney becomes void if a person becomes mentally incapable of managing their affairs. However, the laws of some jurisdictions allow a power of attorney to *continue* or *endure* in the event of physical or mental incapacity. This is called an enduring power of attorney.

A person being considered for a power of attorney should have the following characteristics:

- Have the best interests of your loved one at heart;
- Understand their wishes and values;
- Be willing to make decisions in keeping with those wishes and values;
- Be available and able to address bills and financial needs; and,
- Be able to deal sensitively with any family tensions or dynamics that may arise.

REPRESENTATION AGREEMENT

A representation agreement allows for the appointment of a legal representative to handle personal care and healthcare decisions, as well as routine financial matters if your loved one is unable to make them on their own. The representative cannot be someone who is paid to provide personal or healthcare to your loved one or who is an employee of a facility providing those services, unless that person is your loved one's child, parent or spouse.

The representation agreement creates a contract between your loved one and their representative. This type of agreement sometimes includes the identification of a monitor – another person to help ensure that the representative fulfills their duties, which include consulting with your loved one to determine their wishes or instructions.

LIVING WILL

A living will – also called an advance directive or an advanced healthcare directive – is a legal document that identifies a person's wishes for medical treatments to prolong or sustain life in the event that a person is not able to speak for themselves. It specifies which treatments a person does or does not want to receive in such an event. For example, a living will can be used to request that artificial life supports be withheld or discontinued if a physician determines that a person's condition is terminal, with no hope of recovery. A living will can help take the pressure off of family members concerning medical decisions by identifying your loved one's personal care wishes.

If your loved one is considering a living will, it is a good idea to work with a lawyer to prepare the document, since requirements vary by jurisdiction. A living will and a power of attorney are frequently included in estate planning packages prepared by lawyers with estate planning expertise. Together these documents can help provide comprehensive guidance about your loved one's wishes for medical care. Both documents only apply while your loved one is alive, and cease to be effective upon death.

DO NOT RESUSCITATE ORDER

A do not resuscitate (DNR) order is another kind of advance directive. It is a legal document instructing medical professionals not to perform lifesaving measures if a person's heart stops or if they stop breathing. Some terminally ill people prefer not to receive aggressive resuscitation efforts. A DNR order can be added to a person's medical chart to inform doctors that the person does not want to be resuscitated.

It is very important that this document be signed by your loved one in order for it to be valid. An unsigned DNR order is not enforceable, and may result in unwanted resuscitation efforts, since medical professions in many jurisdictions are legally bound to attempt resuscitation and transport a patient to a hospital unless there is a signed DNR form.

ORGAN OR TISSUE DONATION

Your loved one may wish to consider donating their organs or tissues upon death. It's possible that even if the organs can't be used, tissues such as corneas and heart valves still can be. Donated organs and tissues must be removed soon after death or they cannot be transplanted.

Organ and tissue donation registration is handled differently in each jurisdiction. Some jurisdictions use donor cards, some use drivers' licences, while others have registries. Talk with your loved one's family doctor or medical specialist for further information if your loved one is considering organ or tissue donation.

WHOLE BODY DONATION FOR MEDICAL EDUCATION OR RESEARCH

Your loved one may wish to support teaching and research activities at a medical school by considering whole body donation, to help with the training of professionals in health-related disciplines. Most whole body donations must be arranged ahead of time, and each research facility has different rules and procedures. It is important to be aware that not all bodies are accepted. For information about whole body donation, consider contacting the coroner's office or a large medical research facility near you, such as a university.

CHOOSING WHERE TO DIE

Allowing your loved one to choose where to die can provide them with a sense of comfort and some element of control in their final days.

- **Home** – Some people prefer to die at home in a familiar setting. Home care services or hospice care may be available to assist in making this option possible. If your loved one wishes to die at home, you will need to talk with your physician or hospice team about what arrangements must be made at the time of death (see *Chapter 7: When Death Occurs*). Be aware that some family members may have difficulty visiting or living in a home where a family member has died.
- **Hospital** – It may not be possible to manage your loved one's physical symptoms and treatments at home. Having doctors and nurses available at all times in a hospital may be preferable. Hospital beds may also be available for patients waiting to get into a nursing home or hospice facility.
- **Hospice facility** – A hospice facility looks after people who need care at the end stage of a terminal illness. The focus is on improving the quality of the patient's remaining life by providing comfort and relieving suffering. Hospice rooms are often decorated to create a more welcoming environment than a hospital room, but are not intended for longer-term stays.

- **Nursing home** – A nursing home offers a care option for people in need of longer-term care who are not yet at the end stage of a terminal illness.

There may be costs associated with each of the options mentioned above. Consider discussing these options and the associated referral processes with the family doctor caring for your loved one.

PRESERVING MEMORIES

Caring for a terminally ill loved one can be a time to reflect on life – a time to remember special moments together, to capture memories, to consider family histories. It is often with much regret that people turn their minds to preserving memories only after a loved one passes away, when questions remain unanswered. In the midst of the medical and emotional challenges of illness, exploring and preserving memories can serve as a touch point – a source of comfort as well as a legacy to pass down to future generations.

There are many options for preserving memories. Scrapbooks are a popular means of gathering photos and mementos together. Computer scrapbook programs are available for digitally scanning, recording and organizing photos and documents. These programs make it easier to share material electronically with family and friends.

Audio and video recordings offer another means of capturing and preserving the memories of your loved one. Some people may be uncomfortable appearing on a video recording, particularly if their illness has taken a toll on their physical appearance. Both types of recordings create a permanent record of your loved one's voice – capturing their speech patterns, inflections, warmth and humour. Be sure to check the functioning of any equipment you choose to use, such as the sound quality of the microphone on a tape or video recorder, prior to making any recordings in order to avoid disappointment.

Using an interview format for an audio or video recording can provide a neutral framework for drawing out memories and favourite stories. The interview can be framed using basic biographical details (e.g., family background, childhood, schooling, etc.), or can be based on the things at the center of your loved one's life - such as relationships, interests, hope and dreams. Music and photos can also be used in an interview to help bring back memories of favourite activities, people, places and events.

A journal can provide another means of capturing memories for people who are unable to communicate verbally, or are perhaps not comfortable talking about their thoughts and feelings. A journal allows more time for reflection than an audio or video recording. It can also provide a more comfortable means of expressing things that might be difficult to convey in person.

Preserving your loved one's memories is important for a variety of reasons. Beyond the value of their medical history - which can help inform the medical care of other family members - their memories can provide a sense of belonging, of traditions and stories that bind generations together. Learning about a person's upbringing can shed light on their choices in life and their relationships. Collecting and preserving these memories offers an opportunity to connect with your loved one – to convey the value of the person's experiences and memories. It may also provide them with a much needed opportunity to express unspoken emotions and feelings.

CHAPTER 6

Advance Planning of Arrangements After Death

Life isn't a matter of milestones, but of moments.

Rose Kennedy

Planning in advance for arrangements after death gives your loved one time to consider how they want to be remembered and honoured. It can help remove some of the emotional burden on surviving family and friends. Pre-paying some of the costs may help reduce the financial burden. In some cases, advance planning can also save money. Taking the time to compare prices at several funeral homes may help reduce costs.

It is not recommended to put funeral or memorial service plans in a will, since the arrangements may need to be made before the will can be read. The following section provides some ideas for your loved one to consider when choosing and documenting their preferences for arrangements following their death. One of the first choices to consider is whether your loved one wishes to be buried or cremated.

ARRANGEMENTS FOR THE BODY

Burial

A burial involves placing the remains of your loved one in the ground, usually in a churchyard or cemetery. Some people choose to pre-purchase grave space, often purchasing more than one space to allow for the future burial of a spouse and/or children. Burial fees vary, and may include costs for purchasing the grave, opening or digging the grave, and removing or replacing existing memorials.

A body is usually buried in a casket. Prices for caskets vary widely, and can range from a few hundred dollars to tens of thousands of dollars. Personal items such as photographs or letters may also be placed in the casket prior to burial.

Eco-friendly burial

A green burial or natural burial is an option that involves wrapping the body in a natural shroud such as hemp cloth and placing it in a casket or urn made from materials that are non-toxic and readily biodegradable, allowing the body to naturally decompose. This option reduces the consumption of resources (e.g., chemical preservation, metal casket, etc.) and the environmental impact of the burial.

A natural burial ground often uses living memorials such as native trees, shrubs or plants, or an engraved flat stone native to the area to mark the location of the grave. Natural or green burial cemeteries are available in many countries throughout the world. Organizations such as the Centre for Natural Burial or the Green Burial Council can assist with locating a green burial provider.

Promession

Another relatively new and ecologically-conscious method for caring for the body is called promession. This method was invented in Sweden and involves freeze drying the body, reducing it to a fine powder which decomposes naturally. Metals in the powdered remains are removed and recycled. The remaining powder is then buried in a biodegradable casket at a depth of less than 2 metres where it will disintegrate within 6 to 12 months.

Cremation

Cremation is a process that uses intense heat to reduce the body to bone fragments, which are then crushed or ground into ashes. The cremated remains weigh between four to eight pounds and can be scattered, placed in a box or urn and kept at home, placed in a columbarium (a structure in a memorial garden designed to store cremated remains) or buried in the ground. Inurnment involves the placement of cremated remains in an urn which is then placed in a niche, crypt, grave or other location in a cemetery. Arrangements can be made to have the remains of a body cremated after organ or body donation. Cremation is generally a less expensive option than a burial.

It is usually a requirement that the body be cremated in a container. Most funeral homes offer an inexpensive container for this purpose. However, some people choose to be cremated in an expensive casket. It is important to inform a crematory if the body has a pacemaker or other metal implants, so they can be removed prior to cremation.

TYPES OF SERVICES

Funeral service

A funeral is a service often held within a few days of the death in a funeral home, church or temple. The service can be personalized to be an informal celebration of life, or it can be a more formal service that incorporates traditions or rituals. If a person chooses to be buried, the body is often present during the funeral service. A private viewing of the body can be arranged for close friends and family prior to the service. In some cultures, friends and family say farewell to the deceased and comfort each other by holding a wake – a ceremony where the body is laid out the night before a funeral, often in the house of the deceased. A committal service (see below) sometimes follows a funeral service.

Memorial service, or celebration of life

A memorial service is generally held without the body, allowing for more flexibility around the timing of the service. This type of service can be held anywhere – at home, in a park, at the graveside, in a church or at a community hall. A memorial service can be personalized, much like a funeral service, to be as simple and informal or elaborate and traditional as desired.

Committal service

A committal or burial service usually takes place at the graveside or where the ashes are to be interred. This type of service is sometimes held after a funeral service or in place of a funeral or memorial service, and is usually briefer than a funeral or memorial service. The burial service may be open to all, or reserved only for immediate family and close friends. The service itself may involve lowering the casket into the ground, or placing the cremated remains in a grave or tomb. Friends and family may be invited to share a special memory and place a flower on the casket or grave.

No service

Some people request that no service be held for them after death. This may be because they are very private people, or are uncomfortable at the thought of people gathering to honour them. Others choose to be recognized in some other way, such as a request for loved ones to share a meal together at a favourite restaurant in their honour.

MEMORIAL SOCIETIES

Some jurisdictions have memorial societies or organizations that can help with advance planning and understanding the options available. In many cases, these organizations offer discounts on arrangements after death with certain funeral homes. A one-time membership fee provides access to preferred pricing on funeral services through contracted funeral service providers, ensuring the availability of reasonably priced funeral arrangements. However, membership in these organizations must be purchased before death. For a small fee, membership is transferable among most of the memorial societies in North America. A list of some of the provincial memorial societies in Canada is included in *Appendix 3*.

Form 15: Pre-planning of Arrangements After Death provides a template for documenting your loved one's preferences. A completed sample is shown below.

Form 15: Pre-planning of Arrangements After Death

A ARRANGEMENTS FOR THE BODY

☐ Burial (indicate requested burial location)

____

Indicate clothing and jewellery to be worn, along with any personal items to be placed in the casket

____

☑ Cremation (indicate where ashes should be scattered, buried or preserved)

Ashes to be cremated after organ donation and buried in a simple box with marble memorial stone in Lasting Memories Memorial Garden in Elizabethtown

☑ Yes, there is a pacemaker or metal implant (describe implant)

Metal pin in left ankle from when I broke my ankle 5 years ago

☑ Organ or body donation (indicate what arrangements have been made and where the relevant papers are located)

Organs to be donated as per donation form signed when driver's licence renewed. Remains to be cremated after organ donation.

B TYPE OF SERVICE

☑ Funeral ☐ Memorial ☐ Committal ☐ No service

☐ Other ________________________________

C LOCATION OF SERVICE

☐ Church or temple ________________________________

☑ Funeral home *Lasting Memories Funeral Home in Elizabethtown*

☐ Other ________________________________

D	MUSIC TO BE PLAYED OR SUNG
	List the hymns, chants, songs or other music to be included in the service. Include the names of any preferred singers or musicians. 1. Hymn - Amazing Grace, Singer / Pianist - Cindy Schellenberg 2. Song - With Eagles Wings, Singer / Guitarist - Tony Ladner
E	READINGS
	List favourite scriptures, readings, poems, etc. to be read during the service. Include the names of any preferred readers. 1. Scripture - Psalm 23, Reader - James Wilson 2. Poem - I am not here, Reader - Marion Jones
F	EULOGY
	Identify the names of preferred people to deliver the eulogy. 1. Larry Smith - son-in-law 2. Maureen Graylor - best friend
G	FLOWERS AND DONATIONS
☐	Flowers appreciated for immediate family.
☑	No flowers please. Monetary donations appreciated for: 1. Cancer Society
H	PRE-PLANNING ARRANGEMENTS
☑	Yes, pre-planning arrangements have been made (identify memorial society or funeral home and location of paperwork): Joined Dignity Memorial Society. Paperwork in top left drawer of desk in den. Funeral arrangements (cremation, burial spot for ashes and marble memorial) pre-paid with Lasting Memories Funeral Home in Elizabethtown.
☐	No arrangements have been made.

I	OTHER INSTRUCTIONS OR INFORMATION
	- Favourite piano music by Georgina Winstanley to be played during prelude and postlude. - A bottle of Hautvillers champagne to be shared by immediate family members after my ashes have been buried to honour my memory.

TALKING THINGS THROUGH

Managing the time that remains when a loved one is dying is an incredibly challenging process. Some of the activities that need to be undertaken can be upsetting. However, the task of honouring their wishes after death becomes much more difficult if no conversations have taken place, or if no direction has been given. This can result in family conflicts and additional heartache.

Your loved one may wish to sit down with appropriate family members, friends or advisors to talk about their final wishes and directives, to discuss important documents and information, and to clarify their preferences for where to die and for the arrangements after death. Some people may find this suggestion too difficult. Others may view this as an important contribution– a way to provide closure and peace of mind. Each person and circumstance is unique. Consider what best meets the needs of your loved one.

Decision-making meeting

One option for talking things through involves holding a decision-making meeting with family members, close friends and the medical professionals involved. The purpose of the meeting is to talk openly and honestly about your loved one's illness and about decisions that need to be made in the time that remains, in order to develop a comprehensive plan.

The meeting format, described by Dr. David Kuhl in his book entitled "What Dying People Want: Practical Wisdom for the End of Life," can provide a framework for addressing many of the issues that were discussed in Part I of this book. The meeting involves a five-step process:

1. **Organize the meeting** – Work with your loved one to identify the people they want to attend the meeting. Ask someone with good facilitation skills to lead the meeting. The facilitator can explain the purpose of the meeting, raise issues that might be difficult for your loved one to bring up on their own, and ensure that key decisions are addressed.

2. **Discuss the medical information** – It's helpful for the significant people in your loved one's life to hear firsthand about the diagnosis, symptoms, treatment options and life expectancy. This also provides an opportunity for your loved one to ask for help if they feel they need assistance dealing with the healthcare system on matters such as getting additional information, arranging and attending appointments or seeking another medical opinion.

3. **Identify preferences** – This step involves clarifying your loved one's choices. It includes everything from their preferences for medical treatment to their final wishes and directives. A suggested list of topics to be discussed is identified below:

    - Alternative treatment options
    - Preferred treatment plan
    - Communication with healthcare team
    - Financial assistance
    - Care facilities
    - Last will
    - Power of attorney
    - Advance directives, e.g., living will
    - Organ or body donation
    - Choice of where to die
    - Arrangements after death

4. **Consider quality of life** – At this point, your loved one is given an opportunity to talk about what gives meaning to their life, and to describe the quality of life they hope to experience in the time that remains, on a variety of levels – physically, emotionally, mentally, spiritually, financially and socially.

5. **Assess practical considerations** – Specific actions are identified to help your loved one realize their preferences and achieve their quality-of-life goals. Tasks may include making arrangements for a trip, exploring options for care facilities or identifying sources of financial assistance. A volunteer is identified for each action item, along with a deadline for each task. The facilitator is responsible for setting up a follow-up meeting to check on progress on the action items and to see whether priorities have changed.

The meeting format presented above is one option for framing the issues that need to be discussed when a loved one is facing a life-threatening illness. Having a facilitator can help relieve the pressure when raising some of the difficult issues. The end result can be the creation of a community of caring created specifically to support your loved one, as well as a clear understanding of their wishes for the time that remains and for arrangements after death.

Part Two
What Happens Now

Honouring a Loved One after Death

CHAPTER 7

When Death Occurs

We shall find peace.
We shall hear the angels,
We shall see the sky sparkling with diamonds.
Anton Chekhov

A loved one is close to death. What do you do now?

Part II addresses what happens when death occurs. It walks you through the decisions and tasks that need to be addressed after your loved one dies, including caring for the body, planning a funeral, dealing with grief and executing a will.

PHYSICAL CHANGES WHEN A PERSON IS CLOSE TO DEATH

Each terminal illness has unique symptoms specific to the disease. However, a series of physical changes commonly occur when a person is nearing death. Changes you may observe in your loved one could include:

- Unresponsiveness
- Increased need for sleep
- Little interest in eating or drinking
- Poor blood circulation resulting in cold hands and feet along with pale bluish or blotchy skin coloring
- Changes in breathing patterns such as rapid shallow breathing or extended periods of time between breaths
- Rattling sounds in the lungs and throat due to a buildup of mucus or fluid
- Loss of bladder and bowel control
- Increased restlessness and agitation
- Mental confusion and disorientation

As the end of life draws near, there are some simple things that you can do to make your loved one more comfortable.

PHYSICAL CHANGE	OFFERING COMFORT AND CARE
Unresponsiveness	Your loved one may still be able to hear you. Remind them in a soothing voice that you are still there. Gestures such as holding or massaging their hands or feet and stroking their face or hair may comfort both you and your loved one.
Little interest in eating or drinking	Have water available if they become thirsty. A straw may make it easier for them to drink. Try a bowl of ice chips that can be sucked to moisten the mouth. Lip balm or a vitamin E ointment can help with dry or cracking lips. If they are unable to swallow easily, swabbing the mouth with a damp sponge can help with hydration.
Cold hands and feet	Use a blanket to keep them warm. If they need immediate warming, put a flannel sheet in the dryer for a few minutes, and wrap their hands and/or feet in it.
Difficulty breathing	Keep your loved one's head raised using pillows or by raising the head of the bed to ease breathing. The doctor may also be able to administer some medication to help with congested breathing.
Loss of bladder and bowel control	Disposable underwear or a catheter (a tube put into the bladder so urine can drain into a specially designed collecting bag) can help your loved one stay clean and dry.
Increased restlessness and agitation	Create a calming and peaceful atmosphere in the room. Play soothing music. Check to make sure that your loved one's clothing is comfortable and that incontinence pads or catheters have not been dislodged. Talk to the doctor about medication if your loved one seems in distress.

THE FINAL MOMENTS

Sometimes it seems as though a loved one is hanging on – waiting for someone to visit or something to be said. Some people choose this time to talk about what they will always remember or will cherish most. Others choose to let go of past conflicts, or give permission for their loved one to let go assuring them that those left behind will be all right. Tears are a natural part of saying goodbye.

When death finally occurs, it can be quite disturbing for those attending the death, even though they may have been dealing with the loved one's terminal illness for some time. Physical signs of death include:

- No breathing
- No heartbeat or pulse
- Eyes fixed in one direction, with enlarged pupils
- Relaxed jaw and slightly open mouth
- Loss of control of bladder and bowel (the sheets or undergarments may be soiled)

CARING FOR THE BODY AFTER DEATH

Once death occurs, the body doesn't have to be moved right away. Family members may choose to spend some time alone with the deceased. Some people wish to embrace their loved one after death. Others choose to hold a farewell ceremony or ritual at the bedside. Consider what will provide comfort and closure for family and friends.

You and other family members present may wish to spend a moment caring for the body of your loved one. Medical staff can be asked to disconnect medical equipment to allow for a more intimate farewell free of tubes and machines. A clean top sheet can be placed on the bed. You may wish to wash your loved one's face or brush their hair.

Some things that you may wish to consider doing immediately after death include:

- Inserting dentures back into the mouth
- Closing the eyes, if they are open, although they may open again.
- Removing any jewellery or rings that are not to remain with the body. You may wish to tape rings that are to be left on to prevent them from slipping off as the muscles relax.
- Preparing wigs or other items that are to accompany the body to the funeral home.

PEOPLE TO CALL AT THE TIME OF DEATH

There are people you may wish to notify when death occurs. It's easier if a list of key contacts has been prepared in advance, since this can be a very emotional time. You may wish to make these phone calls yourself. Consider asking a nurse or close friend to help with this task.

Here is a suggested list of people to contact at the time of death:

- Family doctor or attending physician
- Immediate family members
- Close friends
- Funeral director
- Medical school (for whole body donations)
- Minister or spiritual advisor

Friends and extended family members may also wish to be notified once death occurs. Consider asking a relative or friend to assume responsibility for making these phone calls. Creating an email distribution list is a quick way of notifying large groups of people about the death of a loved one, but may be viewed by some people as impersonal.

REMOVAL OF THE BODY AND PERSONAL BELONGINGS

After you've had an opportunity to say goodbye to your loved one, a doctor or coroner needs to certify that the person is dead. If death occurs in a hospital or hospice, the attending physician will take care of this. If death occurs at home or in a nursing home, call the family doctor. If the death was expected, the doctor should be able to issue the medical certificate giving the cause of death. If the doctor is not available or if your loved one did not have a family doctor, call emergency services and ensure that there is a signed Do Not Resuscitate order by the bedside. Ambulance crews are legally required to administer life-saving treatment unless this type of order is in place.

Once the medical certificate of death has been completed, the body of your loved one will be moved to the hospital mortuary, funeral home or medical school. If the death occurred in a hospital or hospice, the body may be moved temporarily to a morgue while transportation is arranged. The attending nurse or doctor can call the funeral home if one has already been chosen. The funeral home will send a vehicle to pick up the body and take it into their care. If your loved one chose to donate their body to medical education or research, the medical school will arrange transportation. When it comes time for the body to be removed, you may wish to leave the room as this experience can be rather distressing.

If a death occurs in a care facility such as a hospital, hospice or nursing home, family members will be asked to remove the personal belongings of their loved one from the room. Care facilities usually have a set time period for clearing out personal effects. Long-term care facilities may allow up to 24 hours, whereas others may only allow a few hours. Knowing this information beforehand will help you plan ahead for items such as boxes and packing supplies.

Be sure to check bedside tables and closets for all personal effects. With emotions raw and grief weighing heavily, it's easy to forget something. Contact the facility staff if something does get forgotten.

THE DEATH REGISTRATION PROCESS

The medical certificate of death completed by the doctor or local coroner is forwarded to the funeral director, who commonly handles the paperwork involved with a person's death. The following information about the deceased is collected by the funeral director with the assistance of a family member or an adult with knowledge of the facts regarding the death, although information requirements vary by jurisdiction:

- Full name
- Home address
- Marital status (marriage certificate may be required)
- Maiden name (if applicable)
- Occupation
- Date and place of birth (birth certificate may be required)
- Date and place of death
- Names and place of birth of parents
- Healthcare number
- Family doctor
- Social insurance / social security number

This information, along with the medical certification of death, is used to register the death with the appropriate government organizations such as the vital records and registration office of the local public health department. Cause-of-death information gathered from death registrations may be used for medical and health research and for statistical purposes.

Once the death has been registered, a formal death certificate can be issued. An official death certificate or certified copy is needed for dealing with the will and settling the estate. The death certificate is issued by a government official such as a registrar of vital statistics, and usually contains the person's full name, gender, date of death, place of death, place of birth, place of residence, registration number and date of registration.

The process and requirements for registering a death and applying for a death certificate vary by jurisdiction. In some areas, applications for a death certificate can be made online, by mail or fax, or in person. The different application processes may have different service times and differing fees depending on the process selected.

A funeral home may issue a Proof of Death certificate, which can be used to provide confirmation of death to government offices, financial institutions and businesses. This type of certificate can be very helpful if there is a backlog for obtaining a government death certificate.

A permit is required before cremation or a burial can take place. In most cases, the funeral director can help obtain the burial permit. If the death occurred in another jurisdiction, a transit or removal permit may also be required from the jurisdiction where the death occurred.

CHAPTER 8

Funeral Arrangements

What we have once enjoyed we can never lose.
All that we love deeply becomes a part of us.

Helen Keller

You may receive many phone calls and visitors immediately after the death of your loved one. Consider asking a friend to answer the door or telephone and record the messages. A phone message book available at an office supply store can help keep track of the messages. A call log is another option for recording the incoming calls. **Form 16: Phone Call Log** provides a template for keeping track.

ADVANCE PLANNING ARRANGEMENTS

Part I of this book provided advice on advance planning for arrangements after death. Before you begin making funeral arrangements, check whether your loved one made any requests, advance planning or pre-payments for arrangements after death. In some cases, the will may include funeral arrangements. However, it is not recommended to include this type of instruction in a will, since it may not be read until after the funeral, when it is too late to carry out the requests or instructions.

One of the roles of the executor or administrator of a will is to help the family arrange for the funeral (see the section on *Role of the executor*). The following section will help you and/ or the executor of the will to think through the decisions that have to be made, including honouring the wishes of your loved one if they provided some advanced planning requests.

Working through the arrangements after death can be emotionally and physically exhausting. People who have recently lost a loved one can be very vulnerable, and may make decisions on caskets, funeral home services and related expenses that they may later regret. Take a trusted friend or family member with you when making funeral arrangements to help you think through the details and associated costs.

SELECTING A FUNERAL HOME

If no prior arrangements have been made, you may wish to contact a funeral home. Make sure that you select one that is licensed by the local authorities and has a good reputation in the community. The licensing of funeral homes helps to ensure that the facilities meet certain standards and that the provider maintains fair and honest business practices.

You can look for funeral homes in the yellow pages of the phone book or on line. Personal recommendations are helpful, and may be available from a local church, hospital or care facility.

ARRANGEMENTS FOR THE BODY

When death has just occurred, the first step is to arrange for the care of the body. Once you've selected a funeral home, they will send a vehicle to pick up your loved one's body and care for it. Once this is taken care of, it's time to think about burial or cremation. Chapter 6 has some basic information on what's involved with each option.

FUNERAL COSTS

There are three basic categories of funeral costs:

- **Professional service fee** – This fee is not optional, and covers the cost of services common to all funerals, including the services of the funeral home director and attendants, transportation of the body to the funeral home, completing government forms, registering the death, obtaining necessary permits, etc.
- **Optional services** – Optional services might include embalming, coordinating a viewing or wake service, transportation costs for the use of a hearse or limousine, burial or cremation containers, etc.
- **Cash disbursements** – The funeral home may purchase goods and services on your behalf, at your request, such as flowers, catering, the placement of obituary notices or the hiring of a musician.

Funeral homes are in business to make money. It pays to shop around, if you have time, since the professional service fee costs may vary significantly between funeral homes. Also, don't be afraid to ask questions.

Funerals are expensive. A very basic funeral can cost $1,000, with more elaborate funerals costing well over $10,000. The National Funeral Directors Association of the United States estimated that the average cost of an adult funeral with burial in 2006 was $6,195. Cremation is generally a less expensive option. If you choose to have a funeral with burial, consider purchasing an affordable casket, since the casket is essentially a box that will end up being buried in the ground.

In Canada, many provinces require funeral providers to disclose all costs ahead of time. In the United States, funeral providers are required by federal law to provide a statement detailing all costs of the funeral goods and services that you select.

Form 17: Estimating Funeral Costs provides a template to help you work through an estimate. A completed sample is shown below.

Form 17: Funeral Cost Estimate

Professional Service Fees		
Funeral director and staff	$	1,500
Optional Services		
Embalming / cremation=> *cremation*	$	650
Other preparations of the body		
Viewing / wake service - facility and staff fee		
Funeral / memorial service - facility and staff fee	$	550
Cemetery / graveside service		
Hearse		
Limousine	$	200
Casket / cremation urn => *metal burial urn*	$	175
Burial plot / urn vault => *urn burial site*	$	1,700
Memorial / headstone => *bronze / granite burial site marker*	$	150
Cash Disbursements		
Floral arrangements	$	150
Catering	$	400
Musician	$	125
Other => officiant	$	225
TOTAL	**$**	**5,875**

PLANNING A FUNERAL SERVICE

In *Chapter 5: Advance Planning of Arrangements After Death*, three types of services were described: a funeral service, a memorial service or celebration of life, and a committal service. Each can be personalized based on the wishes of your loved one and those of the surviving family members.

Here are some ideas to consider if you choose to hold a service.

- **Location** – A good starting point for choosing a location is figuring out how many people you think will attend the service. For a small family gathering, a chapel in a funeral home may be suitable. For larger groups, a church or temple may be more appropriate. For very large groups, a community hall or auditorium may be needed. Remember to mention the time and location of the service in the obituary (refer to the next section on *Writing an Obituary*).
- **Viewing, or wake** – If you choose burial, you may wish to consider holding a special gathering in a funeral home, at the home of the deceased or at a church to allow for the viewing of the body in advance of the service. Participation is often limited to immediate family and friends, and is meant as a time of both mourning and celebrating the life of a loved one.
- **Officiant** – You may wish to lead the service yourself; however, a service can be very emotional and difficult to face. It may be more practical to ask a minister or family friend to help plan and lead the service. This person is sometimes called a funeral officiant. In the United States, there is the American Association of Funeral Officiants. Choose someone who will support you and help you express your wishes to honour your loved one.
- **Music** – The selection of music to be played at the service is an opportunity to reflect the interests and personality of your loved one. You may wish to play one of their favourite songs or albums using the sound system in the chapel or hall before and after the service. Hiring musicians, or giving family or friends the opportunity to play or sing a song can be a way of helping those close to you to show their love and support.
- **Readings** – Consider whether your loved one had a favourite poem, short story or passage of scripture. Many websites or books feature readings or reflections that you may wish to incorporate into the service.
- **Eulogy** – A eulogy is a speech given during a funeral or memorial service to help people remember the person who has died – who they were, what they did and what they enjoyed about life. It is usually given by someone who knew the person well. The eulogy may contain an overview of their life, their interests and achievements, favourite poems or quotes, and humorous or touching memories.

- **Flowers** – Flowers are often placed at the front of the chapel or meeting room during a funeral or memorial service. Again, this is an opportunity to honour the preferences of your loved one by including a favourite plant, flower or arrangement. If you are holding a committal service, you may wish to distribute flowers to each of those attending, with a request that they place a flower on the casket after sharing something about the person who has died.
- **Photographs / memorial** – Photos or a collage of memories and stories can be displayed in the chapel or hall to celebrate the life of your loved one. Another option is to create a photo slideshow that can be played before or after the service.
- **Memorial keepsake** – A keepsake can be created and handed out at the service. One option is to feature a treasured photo of your loved one in a small booklet or folded piece of paper. The inside of the keepsake could include the order of service, a favourite poem or quote, or a copy of the obituary.
- **Donations** – If you have requested donations to a charity in lieu of flowers, it's helpful to provide information during the service on how to donate. This information might be included in an announcement, in the memorial keepsake, on a sign in the lobby or it could be handed out by ushers when seating guests. If possible, include the donation information in the obituary.
- **Guest register** – A guest register is usually placed at the entrance to the service to record the names of guests. A friend or family member may wish to stand by the register before and after the service to alert guests to the register and to invite them to sign.
- **Ushers / greeters** – Guests are normally seated by ushers or greeters who can hand out an order of service or keepsake, help guests find seats and assist with the set up and coordination of any slide shows, CD's or music to be played during the service.
- **Reception** – Holding a reception after the service provides an opportunity for family and friends to celebrate the life of your loved one and to support each other. Funeral homes often have a room that can accommodate a reception immediately after the service, and can also arrange for catering. Family and friends may wish to provide baking and assorted appetizers for the reception as a way of contributing to the service. Request that the officiant or a family friend coordinate this. You have enough on your mind already.

Form 18: Planning a Service provides a template to help you develop a plan. The completed example below is for a funeral service, but the form could be adapted for a memorial or committal service.

Form 18: Planning a Service

LOCATION	
Address:	Pleasant Memories Funeral Home
Contact:	Francis Dryden
Tel # / Email:	1-800-364-9997; fdryden@pleasant memories.com
Date / Time:	Saturday, March 15 at 2:00pm
Seating capacity:	125 people
OFFICIANT	
Name:	Reverend James Wilson
Tel # / Email:	896-7828; jwilson@mail.ca
MUSIC	
Before the service:	CD, Georgina Winstanley, Memories album
During the service:	Hymn – Great is Thy Faithfulness
	Special music – With Eagles' Wings
	Song – There is Hope
After the service:	CD, Instrumental album, Nature Sings
Musician:	Tony Ladner
Tel # / Email:	tladner@musicians.com
READINGS	
Poem:	I am not there
Scripture:	Psalm 23
EULOGY	
Delivered by:	Reginald Arnaud
Tel # / Email:	rarnaud@mail.com

FLOWERS	
Flower shop:	*Flowers on Broadway*
Tel # / Email:	*1-800-987-6543*
Flowers requested:	*Red rose arrangement on the casket; Two spring flower arrangements for the front of the church*

PHOTOGRAPHS / MEMORIAL	
Photos:	*Head shot photo at age 40 to be featured at the front of the church and in the memorial keepsake*
Memorial:	*Collage of casual photos and favourite things (e.g., rabbit Thumper, harp, family gatherings, volunteer work, etc.)*
Placement:	*Head shot photo at front of church; collage in lobby of church*

MEMORIAL KEEPSAKE	
Format:	*3 ½" x 5" folded card stock*
Photo:	*Head shot photo at age 40*
Content:	*Front cover: head shot; Inside pages: order of service; Back cover: picture of eagle soaring*

DONATIONS	
Charity:	*Breast cancer society*
How to donate:	*Donation forms to be distributed by ushers*

GUEST REGISTER	
Type of register:	*Blue with tree imprint*
Register attendant:	*Donna Arnaud, Niece*
Tel # / Email:	*darnaud@pacifica.net*

USHERS / GREETERS	
Name:	Dougray Arnaud; Nephew
Tel # / Email:	425-8976
Name:	Bradley Henrickson; Nephew
Tel # / Email:	785-4234
RECEPTION	
Location:	Pleasant Memories Funeral Home
Catering contact:	Annie Bowden; Catering is Us
Tel # / Email:	555-4432; cateringisus@gmail.com

The information in the "Planning a Service" form becomes the basis for an order of service for a funeral, memorial or committal service. **A sample order of service** for a funeral is shown below.

Sample: Funeral Order of Service

FUNERAL ORDER OF SERVICE
Prelude
Welcome and introductory remarks
Prayer
Hymn / song – Great is Thy Faithfulness
Reading – Psalm 23
Special music – With Eagles' Wings
Poem – I am not there
Eulogy
Hymn / song – There is Hope
Reflection
Closing prayer or blessing
Postlude

WRITING AN OBITUARY

An obituary is a notice or announcement of a person's death. It often includes a short overview of their life, highlighting accomplishments as well as the impact the person had on their family, friends and community. It also provides details of any services to take place.

Most newspapers charge by the word when placing obituaries. You may wish to confirm the costs before you begin writing. Some obituaries include a photograph, although there is usually an extra cost associated with this.

Obituaries are often sent to local newspapers to advise friends and family of funeral or memorial service arrangements. You'll want to think about the timing of the obituary so that it runs a few days prior to the funeral or memorial service. Obituaries may also be forwarded to newspapers in areas where your loved one formerly lived. Some request that the obituary be forwarded to other publications such as professional journals.

The following outline can help guide your thoughts when writing an obituary.

1. **Introduction** – Contains basic information such as the person's full name, age, and date and place of death.
2. **Next of kin** – Acknowledges surviving family members and important relationships such as parents, children, grandchildren, etc. Surviving relatives are sometimes mentioned by name, with the partner or spouse of the family member identified in parentheses. If there are many surviving family members, the obituary may acknowledge groups of family members by noting that the deceased had 10 grandchildren, 6 nephews, etc. Special friends or companions are sometimes included in this section.
3. **Life overview** – Includes highlights and accomplishments of the person's life such as their occupation, education, special achievements, volunteer work, military service, special interests, hobbies or awards.
4. **Funeral arrangements** – Identifies funeral, memorial or committal service arrangements including time and location, as well as information on any requests for charitable donations in lieu of flowers.

Form 19: Writing an Obituary provides a template. A sample obituary is shown below.

Form 19: Obituary

OBITUARY
HERIOT – Quentin James
May 19, 1944 – October 17, 2009
It is with deepest sadness we announce the passing of Quentin James Heriot at Qualicum Hospice at the age of 65 after a brief battle with cancer. Predeceased by his parents Lynn and Raymond, he will be dearly missed by his wife of 43 years Kathy, daughter Susan (Rodney), son Peter (Isabelle), sister Sherry (Bill), brother Leonard (Marion), niece Mary, nephew Ryan and grandchildren Brandon, Jennifer and Samantha. A loyal and devoted husband, Quentin took great pride and joy in his family. He will be fondly remembered by his many friends and co-workers at Hyacinthe Lumber, and by the countless friends and neighbours he touched with his kindness, generosity and sense of humour. A funeral service will be held at 2:00pm on October 24, 2009 at Ocean View Church, 637 Hope Road, Open Bay. In lieu of flowers, donations may be made in Quentin's name to your local hospice society.

CHAPTER 9

Grief and Grieving

The angels are always near to those who are grieving, to whisper to them that their loved ones are safe in the hand of God.

Eileen Elias Freeman

With the many decisions that have to be made immediately after someone dies, it may be days or weeks before you begin to fully understand the impact of your loss.

FIVE STAGES OF GRIEF

The five stages of dying in Part I of this book can also be used to make sense of the grief experienced by those who have lost a loved one. These stages are based on the work of Elisabeth Kübler-Ross and are part of a process of healing.

- **Denial** – In grieving the loss of a loved one, a person may have trouble accepting that death has occurred. They may still feel as though the person will walk through the door at any moment. Their mind may have difficulty processing the truth. This first stage of grieving can help a person survive the loss of a loved one. A sense of numbness, shock and disbelief can help a person cope initially.
- **Anger** – As denial fades, the reality of the loss begins to sink in. Anger may surface towards your loved one for leaving you alone or for not putting their affairs in order. You may feel angry at the doctors for not doing more or at God for allowing your loved one to die. Anger is a natural reaction and can be an expression of underlying pain. It is important to find ways to release your anger without hurting yourself or others through exercise, screaming into a pillow or hitting a punching bag.
- **Bargaining** – Bargaining after the death of a loved one may take the form of "what if" – a reliving of the choices that occurred before death. "What if we had caught the tumour sooner? What if we had chosen a more aggressive treatment?" Bargaining is one means of trying to restore order to the chaos of life after the death of a loved one.
- **Depression** – Once the reality of death hits home, a deeper level of grief and depression may occur. Intense sadness and hopelessness may overshadow the activities of each day. Simple tasks like getting

out of bed or preparing a meal may seem overwhelming. Depression is a normal part of grieving. If depression lasts for an extended period of time, it's important to seek medical assistance.

- **Acceptance –** The final stage of grief involves accepting the reality that a loved one is physically gone – that life has been forever changed. It involves acknowledging all that has been lost, and learning to live with that loss. A person may demonstrate acceptance by exploring ways to remember their loved one and commemorate the loss. Reaching a point of acceptance may take days, months or years.

Grieving is a very personal process, unique to each individual. Just as with the five stages of dying, the stages of grief may not be experienced in a linear fashion. You may go back and forth between some of the stages. The stages model describes what you might be experiencing, rather than prescribing a set pattern or map to be followed.

Other theories have suggested that people go through phases in the process of mourning, or work through a series of tasks (e.g., creating a sustained emotional connection with a loved one), as part of the grieving process. However, the grieving experience is complex and diverse. Each person's experience of loss and grief varies considerably. Taking the time to grieve, in your own way, will allow you to explore and hopefully understand your feelings, form new relationships and begin to live again.

THE PHYSICAL AND EMOTIONAL EFFECTS OF GRIEF

Grief affects each person differently. In an article entitled *The Physical and Emotional Effects of Grief*, Brook Noel describes some of the symptoms that you may be feeling as you grieve the death of your loved one.

- **Exhaustion** – One of the most common symptoms is exhaustion. Day-to-day activities suddenly seem overwhelming. Take time to rest and grieve.
- **Distraction** – It may seem difficult to focus even on the most basic of tasks. Recognize that you need to slow down and lower your expectations of yourself.
- **Waves of sadness** – Grief often surfaces unexpectedly. Uncontrollable moments of sadness are normal, especially over the first three to six months.
- **Physical symptoms** – Grief also has a physical effect on our bodies. Common symptoms include:

  - Aches and pains
  - Sleep difficulties
  - Numbness
  - Restlessness
  - Disorientation
  - Migraines or headaches
  - Poor appetite or overeating
  - Shakiness or trembling
  - Shortness of breath
  - Dizziness

- Dry mouth
- Crying
- Upset stomach
- Weakness

- **Withdrawal** – Some people withdraw and become numb, unable to participate in activities that they once enjoyed. This is one way that the human body protects you from overwhelming emotions.
- **Impulsiveness** – Taking unnecessary risks or compulsively pursuing activities is an emotional response to grief. Monitoring your behaviour for impulsive decisions is particularly important during the first year.
- **Surreal thinking** – For some, the concept of time disappears and everything becomes a blur. It can feel as though you're a spectator watching a play, or experiencing a bad dream. This is another way that your body is coping with loss.

In addition to the symptoms Noel describes above, you may feel anger, guilt or regret. If any of the symptoms noted above persist or concern you, consider seeking advice from your doctor or a grief counsellor.

COPING WITH GRIEF

Grief is a natural response to the death of a loved one. The grieving process may take months for some, and years for others. As your journey through grief unfolds, here are some ideas that may help you cope.

- **Talking** – Talk with a friend, family member, therapist or counsellor. Don't be afraid to let people know what you need or would find helpful.
- **Spiritual comfort** – Seek comfort through religious traditions or spiritual activities that are meaningful to you such as mourning rituals, praying or meditating.
- **Support group** – Join a support group with others who have experienced a similar loss.
- **Counselling** – Speak with a therapist or grief counsellor to help you work through your feelings and emotions.
- **Journaling** – Write in a journal to express your thoughts and feelings.
- **Preserving memories** – Create a scrapbook or photo album to celebrate and remember your loved one's life.
- **Self-care** – Take care of your body by getting enough sleep, eating properly and exercising. Avoid using alcohol or drugs to cope with grief.

SIGNS OF UNHEALTHY GRIEVING

It's important to watch for signs of unhealthy grieving. In the companion workbook to *I Wasn't Ready to Say Goodbye,* Brook Noel and Pamela Blair identify the following signs of someone suffering from unhealthy grief.

- **Prolonged avoidance** – Avoiding friends and family for prolonged periods of time (more than three weeks).
- **Poor self-care** – Having problems taking care of basic physical needs like sleep, food and hygiene.

- **Prolonged denial** – Continuing to deny the death of your loved one months later by keeping all their belongings as they used to be, maintaining routines such as cooking for them.
- **Self-destructive thoughts** – Having persistent or obsessive thoughts of harming yourself.
- **Displaced anger** – Experiencing anger that is causing harm to others either personally or professionally.
- **Prolonged depression or anxiety** – Experiencing ongoing depression or anxiety that gets in the way of daily activities.
- **Self-medication** – Numbing your grief through the excessive use of food, alcohol or drugs.

If you are experiencing any of the signs of unhealthy grief, seek help from a doctor, support group, counsellor or therapist.

HELPING CHILDREN COPE WITH GRIEF

Children also experience grief. Their reactions to the death of a loved one will vary depending on a variety of factors including their age, personality, relationship to the person who died, and on the reactions of the people around them. In the article "*Helping Children Cope with Death,*" Kirsti Dyer identifies a number of practical things to help a child or adolescent cope with the death of a loved one.

- **Daily routines** – Continuing daily routines, as much as possible, can be comforting and help a child be able to starting mourning. Try to minimize major changes in their environment (e.g., a new school, a new house).
- **Talking** – Tell them what you are feeling, in a way that is age appropriate. This helps the child understand that it's OK to talk about the death. Allow the child to talk with you about the death and about their feelings. It's important to hear and acknowledge their feelings.
- **Reassurance** – Reassure the child that you are keeping them safe and watching over them. Regularly express your love and acceptance of them.
- **Family rituals** – Give the child an opportunity to participate in family rituals to remember their loved one. This might include attending the funeral, taking flowers to the cemetery, or planning a special activity on the anniversary of the death.
- **Simple explanations** – Answer any questions honestly and directly, using concrete words such as died and death. Using terms like "passed away" or "went to sleep" can be confusing to a child.
- **Expressing grief** – Help the child discover positive ways to express their grief such as reading stories that talk about death and dying, drawing, or writing a letter to their loved one.

There are a number of excellent books available to help you talk with a child about death and dying. See *Appendix 2* for a listing of resources to help children understand and express their grief.

CHAPTER 10

Settling the Estate

To live in hearts we leave behind
Is not to die.

Thomas Campbell

An estate is made up of the assets or items a person owns at death, such as real estate or jewellery, minus the personal debts or liabilities owed. The distribution of an estate is documented in a will – a signed legal document that clarifies how your loved one wants their assets distributed upon death and who is responsible for administering or executing the will (see *Chapter 5: Final* Wishes and Advance Directives for considerations when drawing up a will).

WHAT HAPPENS IF THERE IS NO WILL

If your loved one died without a valid will, as determined by local laws, they are considered to have died intestate – without a will. In these circumstances, local statutory regulations, called intestacy rules, will determine how the assets are to be distributed. These rules historically focus on relationships by blood (e.g., children, brothers or sisters) or by marriage (e.g., spouse).

Intestacy rules vary by jurisdiction. For example, some jurisdictions have laws that protect a spouse's interest in the family home of the estate even if someone dies intestate. In other jurisdictions, common-law spouses do not receive automatic rights to property.

Without a will, the affairs of your loved one may require the appointment of an administrator by the courts. The cost of administering an estate is often higher without a will. Additional costs may include legal fees as well as the posting of a bond to ensure the assets in the estate are not mismanaged by the administrator. If there are children under the age of majority, the courts will appoint a legal guardian, who may not be the person your loved one wanted to assume this role.

ADMINISTERING THE WILL

It is much easier to honour the wishes of your loved one if they have documented in a will how they want their assets distributed. Ideally, you already know the location of the will and are aware of its contents. If you are unsure whether your loved one had a will, you may wish to check with their lawyer. The executor or person designated to manage the estate should receive the original will so they can carry out their responsibilities.

ROLE OF THE EXECUTOR

The executor is responsible for managing and distributing a person's assets in accordance with the deceased's final wishes as expressed in the will and according to local laws. Some jurisdictions use different titles for this function, such as estate trustee or liquidator. If you are serving as the executor of the will, you may wish to seek legal counsel concerning any personal liability associated with performing the duties of an executor.

Working through an estate can take a considerable amount of time, depending on its size and complexity. The following section provides an overview of the key actions to be taken by an executor.

Assist with the funeral arrangements

- Organize or assist with the funeral according to the wishes of the deceased, if they were made known in advance.

Locate important documents

- Obtain the original Death Certificate and arrange for certified copies.
- Obtain copies of the Proof of Death Certificate from the funeral home, if available.
- Locate the original of the will, any lists or inventories of personal assets and property, and important papers such as deeds and insurance policies. The work of the executor will be made easier if your loved one took the time to review and organize their important documents and information, as discussed in Chapter 4.
- Locate important certificates such as the birth certificate, social insurance or social security card, and marriage certificate. These certificates may be required to establish claims for life insurance or other benefits.
- Determine if the will needs to be probated (see *What is probate?* in the next section for more information), and if so, complete the probate application process in order to obtain court approval and relevant documentation.

Put the financial affairs in order

- Consider seeking legal and financial advice for the management of the estate.
- Determine the immediate financial needs of any dependent family members so that bills and daily expenses can be managed.
- Identify whether there are any assets, such as rental properties, that may require immediate attention.
- Locate all beneficiaries, including charities, and consider whether there are any potential issues such as

beneficiaries who may be disgruntled about the size of their inheritance.

- Open an estate bank account, and transfer any existing bank accounts to the estate account. This will allow for the tracking of all receipts and disbursements related to the estate.
- Cancel accounts and notify relevant organizations (see *Form 20: Accounts / Organizations Checklist*). Using a standard letter to inform organizations of a person's death may help make the process easier (see Form 21 for a template of a notification letter).
  - Cancel the accounts of the deceased person. It can be a rather time-consuming process to track down all of the active accounts, which may include utilities (e.g., hydro, telephone, cable), subscriptions (e.g., newspapers, magazines), health club memberships, credit cards, etc. Other accounts to be cancelled include the deceased's driver's licence, healthcare plan, pension and old age benefits. Reviewing the person's mail and bills may assist you in compiling the list of accounts to be cancelled. Proof of death may required by some organizations in order to cancel an account (see the "Obligations" section of Chapter 4: Important Documents and Information for a template to list and track the accounts).
  - Contact insurance companies requesting benefits payable. Remember to check for insurance policies that are related to credit cards, a mortgage, education funds, etc.
  - Contact the person's employer to determine if there are any pension, life insurance or survivor benefits.
  - Notify federal income security or social security offices and/or the veteran's office if the person served in the armed forces, to cancel any existing benefits and apply for death or survivor benefits payable.
- Develop an inventory of assets (see *Chapter 4: Important Documents and Information*). If an inventory was prepared before death, confirm the accuracy of the list. Assets include everything from real estate and personal property (e.g., jewellery) to investments, life insurance and bank accounts.
- Develop a list of debts or liabilities.

Settle the estate debts

- Advertise for creditors or other interested parties who may have a claim against the estate.
- Settle all legitimate estate debts including credit cards, mortgages and other debt.

File the tax returns

- Consider hiring an accountant to assist with the filing of all relevant tax returns, including any outstanding tax returns for years prior to the date of death, tax returns required for any assets held outside the country, as well as the final tax return.

- Obtain a tax clearance certificate, which protects the executor from any future liability (see *Tax Clearance Certificate* section below for more information). It is important to confirm the process and criteria for issuing the tax clearance certificate, since the requirements vary by jurisdiction.

Distribute the estate assets

- Make a preliminary transfer of assets to the beneficiaries as outlined in the will, reserving enough money to pay any remaining debts, including estate taxes owing, legal, executor or accounting fees, etc.

Wind-up the estate

- File the final tax return for the estate once all debts have been paid and all assets distributed.
- Prepare a final summary of the estate accounts.
- Close the estate bank account.

WHAT IS PROBATE?

Probate refers to the legal process of reviewing a will to determine whether it is valid and authentic, and confirming the authority of the executor named in the will. Probating may be required if there is more than one version of a will. Probate is almost always required by banks, trust companies or other financial institutions as a means of ensuring that the funds are being distributed to the legitimate beneficiaries of an estate, or if a deceased person owned real estate.

Probate requirements vary by jurisdiction. In some states, anyone in the possession of the will of someone who has died must bring the will to the Probate Court for filing. The office responsible for addressing probate requirements may be called the Probate, Surrogate, or Wills and Estate Court.

When a will is submitted to a court to be probated, the estate will be required to pay probate or courts fees. In some jurisdictions, these fees are based on the value of the estate. The probate application form may require a complete listing of all of the assets and property in the estate, including their market value at time of death. Once the court has reviewed and approved the application, a Probate Certificate, a Grant of Probate Document or a Certificate for Administration of the Estate with a Will is issued. This means that the executor can begin to transfer the estate assets in accordance with the will.

ADVERTISING FOR CREDITORS

The executor of the estate may be personally liable for a creditor's claim if the assets of the estate are distributed before the claims of all creditors have been addressed. Advertising for creditors with claims against the estate may protect the estate from any future claims. The advertisement often includes a time limit for the filing of a claim against the estate, for example within 30 days of the date of publication. People who owed money to the deceased are also requested to pay any debts owing to the estate.

Requirements for the content and form of the advertisement vary. Most jurisdictions require the advertisement to run several times in the local newspaper in the area of the deceased's last known address.

Sample: Advertisement for Estate Debtors and Creditors

Oswald Estate

Notice to Debtors and Creditors

All creditors of the Estate of Diedre A. Oswald, deceased, late of Greenfield County, are hereby notified to render their demands to the undersigned according to law, and all persons indebted to the Estate are required to make immediate payment to the undersigned. This 21st day of July, 2010.

Geraldine M. Stuart, Executrix
Estate of Diedre A. Oswald, Deceased
507 Magnolia Blossom Way, Summerfield, BC

ESTATE TAXES

There are currently no estate taxes or succession duties in Canada. However, some jurisdictions, notably the United States, apply taxes on estates. If an asset is left to a spouse or a charitable organization, the estate tax may not apply.

CAPITAL GAINS AND LOSSES

The final tax return for the deceased must take into consideration any capital gains or losses from estate assets. A capital gain is the increase in value of an asset between the time it is bought and the time it is sold. A tax on capital gains commonly applies to the sale of assets like cottages, stock and bonds, as well as land, buildings or equipment used in a business. A capital loss is the decrease in value of an asset between the time it is bought and the time it is sold.

TAX CLEARANCE CERTIFICATE

An estate cannot be fully settled until a final income tax return has been filed and the estate receives a tax clearance certificate. This certificate confirms that the deceased's taxes have been paid in full, and helps protect the executor from any future income tax liability for the estate.

FINANCIAL RECORDS AND ACCOUNTS

Notifying the government of a death

A number of government departments require notification of a death. In Canada, the Service Canada office has all of the forms needed to address federal notifications. The Vital Statistics Agencies in a number of provinces notify Service Canada electronically when a death has occurred. Notification requirements as well as the nearest Service Canada office can be confirmed by calling 1-800-O-CANADA.

In the United States, it is important to notify the Social Security Administration (SSA) office if your loved one was receiving Social Security or Medicare benefits. The funeral director in many cases will take care of this notification. The Social Security number of the deceased is required in order to complete the paperwork. Any Social Security cheques which arrive after death will need to be returned to the SSA. Additional information is available online at www.socialsecurity.gov or by calling the SSA at 1-800-772-1213.

Death benefits

The Canada Pension Plan (CPP) is a national plan administered by the Government of Canada. A person must have paid into the plan in order to be eligible for a one-time lump-sum death benefit payment equal to six months' worth of the deceased's retirement pension, up to a maximum of $2,500.

Several forms must be submitted to notify the Government of a death, and apply for the CPP death benefit.

- **Notification of Death Form** - This form is used to confirm the death of a CPP recipient. This will ensure that any CPP payments are stopped and will prevent an overpayment to your loved one's account.
- **Application for a Canada Pension Plan Death Benefit** – This application must be accompanied by a document confirming proof of death (e.g., certified copy of the death certificate), along with your loved one's social insurance number.

For more information on the CPP death benefit and documents acceptable for proof of death, see www.servicecanada.gc.ca/eforms/forms/isp1200e.pdf.

The Province of Quebec administers a similar plan for workers in Quebec through the Quebec Pension Plan (QPP). Information on the QPP is available at: www.rrq.gouv.qc.ca

In the United States, certain family members may be eligible to receive survivors' benefits, including widows, widowers, children and dependent parents. It is important to apply for survivors' benefits as soon as possible, since in some cases, benefits will be paid from the time you apply rather than the time your loved one died. The benefit amount is based on their earnings before death.

You will be required to provide original or certified copies of the following documents in order to apply for survivors' benefits:

- Proof of death from a funeral home or a death certificate;
- The social security numbers for you and for your loved one;
- Your birth certificate;
- Your marriage certificate if you are a widow or widower; and,
- The name of your bank and your account number so that benefits can be deposited directly into your account.

More information on survivors' benefits is available at: www.socialsecurity.gov/survivorplan.

In addition, a one-time lump-sum death benefit of $255 may be payable to an eligible spouse or child. Survivors must apply for this benefit within two years of the date of death. SSA forms are available online at: www.socialsecurity.gov/online/.

Bank accounts

Official notification requirements may vary depending on the bank. Try calling to confirm each bank's policies and the forms required to close an account after death. Banks generally require an original or certified copy of the person's death certificate.

They will also require documentation of your authority to act on behalf of your loved one. If the account was joint, the other person listed on the account can close it. If it was only in your loved one's name, the account can be closed by the executor of the will. Take documentation with you – like the will if it identifies you as the executor, or a letter from a probate court designating you as the personal representative of the estate. Make sure to also take photo identification, such as a driver's licence or passport.

Life insurance policies

Life insurance claims need to be filed in a timely manner, since policies often include a time limit for filing a claim, normally ranging from 90 days to 12 months. It is the responsibility of the beneficiary or their representative to request payment of a life insurance policy. For policies purchased individually, contact the life insurance agent or the company branch office to file a claim. For group insurance policies such as those purchased through an employer or a union, contact the group benefits administrator.

Generally, proceeds payable from an insurance policy with a named beneficiary do not become part of the estate, and are paid directly to the beneficiary. The life insurance company will require proof of death. Proceeds will usually be available within a matter of weeks, and are paid directly to the named beneficiary. If the estate is named as the beneficiary, estate documentation will be required before any funds are released.

If you are unsure if there is a life insurance policy, or if you are unable to locate one, there are organizations that can perform a search for you – often for a fee. In Canada, there is a voluntary trade association of life and health insurers – the Canadian Life and Health Insurance Association – that can assist with a search. Death benefits are usually paid out very quickly, upon receiving proof of the insured person's death, and are generally not taxable.

Personal Belongings

Once the will has been administered and the distribution of your loved one's assets has taken place, there are often personal belongings that remain – clothing, books, small kitchen appliances, etc. Sorting through these belongings can be a very painful process. Consider asking a friend or a relative to help, or consider sharing some of the items such as housewares, clothing, shoes or accessories with friends who might be honoured to receive something from your loved one.

If you choose not to keep what remains, consider donating the belongings to a not-for-profit organization such as those listed below. Many of these organizations also offer a free pick-up service. Check out their respective websites for examples of acceptable donation items – such as gently used clothing and small household items – and to learn how to prepare your items for donation (e.g., housewares bagged, beds dismantled).

- **Big Brothers Big Sisters (Boys & Girls Clubs)** - Donations picked up from the doorstep or a drop-off bin are sold to Value Village stores, offering low income families inexpensive options, with profits going toward community programs.
- **Habitat for Humanity ReStores -** Non-profit home improvement stores and donation centers that sell new and gently used furniture, home accessories, building materials and appliances to the public at a fraction of the retail price. Proceeds are used to build homes, community and hope, locally and around the world.
- **Charity Thrift Stores** – Donated goods including clothing, household items and furniture are given directly to women and their families or sold at affordable prices to community members to help fund programs for women, hospice, etc.

AFTERWORD

May the road rise up to meet you. May the wind be ever at your back. May the sun shine warm upon your face and the rain fall softly on your fields. And until we meet again, may God hold you in the hollow of his hand.

~Irish Blessing

We spend so much time thinking about living, and so little time preparing for death, even though each of us must face death one day. My hope is that this book has helped you – given you practical ideas on what to think about and work through both before and after the death of your loved one.

My mother passed away in 1998, and yet I still find myself crying on occasion, longing to talk with her – be with her. Losing a loved one leaves its mark – emotions, memories, pain. What will you do with that experience?

I am forever changed by the loss of my mother, by the experience of being by her side on her final journey. I have chosen to write about this experience to honour her and to reach out to all those who must one day walk beside a loved one on their final journey.

With thoughts and prayers,

Jeanne M. Sedun

Form 1: Discussions with Healthcare Professionals

DATE	DOCTOR	COMMENTS	NEXT STEPS

Form 2: Medical Specialists Contact List

SPECIALIST	FUNCTION	ADDRESS	TEL / FAX

Form 3: Medication Schedule

MEDICATION	DOSAGE	DIRECTIONS	PURPOSE	12 AM	2 AM	4 AM	6 AM	8 AM	10 AM	12 PM	2 PM	4 PM	6 PM	8 PM	10 PM

Form 4: Monitoring Health Changes

DATE	TIME	SYMPTOM / REACTION	CIRCUMSTANCE

Form 5: Listing of Key Contacts

NAME	RELATIONSHIP	TELEPHONE	EMAIL

Form 6: Bank Account Information

FINANCIAL INSTITUTION		
ADDRESS		
TEL / FAX / EMAIL		
ACCOUNT TYPE	ACCOUNT NUMBER	OWNERSHIP

FINANCIAL INSTITUTION		
ADDRESS		
TEL / FAX / EMAIL		
ACCOUNT TYPE	ACCOUNT NUMBER	OWNERSHIP

FINANCIAL INSTITUTION		
ADDRESS		
TEL / FAX / EMAIL		
ACCOUNT TYPE	ACCOUNT NUMBER	OWNERSHIP

Form 7: Life Insurance Policy Information

INSURANCE COMPANY	
TYPE OF INSURANCE (Term, Whole Life, Universal)	
POLICY VALUE	
POLICY NUMBER	
BENEFICIARY	
POLICY LOCATION	
INSURANCE AGENT	
TEL / FAX / EMAIL	

INSURANCE COMPANY	
TYPE OF INSURANCE (Term, Whole Life, Universal)	
POLICY VALUE	
POLICY NUMBER	
BENEFICIARY	
POLICY LOCATION	
INSURANCE AGENT	
TEL / FAX / EMAIL	

INSURANCE COMPANY	
TYPE OF INSURANCE (Term, Whole Life, Universal)	
POLICY VALUE	
POLICY NUMBER	
BENEFICIARY	
POLICY LOCATION	
INSURANCE AGENT	
TEL / FAX / EMAIL	

Form 8: Investment Account Information

INVESTMENT FIRM		
INVESTMENT ADVISOR		
ADDRESS		
TEL / FAX / EMAIL		
ACCOUNT TYPE	ACCOUNT NUMBER	OWNERSHIP

INVESTMENT FIRM		
INVESTMENT ADVISOR		
ADDRESS		
TEL / FAX / EMAIL		
ACCOUNT TYPE	ACCOUNT NUMBER	OWNERSHIP

INVESTMENT FIRM		
INVESTMENT ADVISOR		
ADDRESS		
TEL / FAX / EMAIL		
ACCOUNT TYPE	ACCOUNT NUMBER	OWNERSHIP

Form 9: Other Investments

COMPANY		
CONTACT		
TEL / FAX / EMAIL		
DESCRIPTION	POLICY / PLAN #	DOCUMENT LOCATION

COMPANY		
CONTACT		
TEL / FAX / EMAIL		
DESCRIPTION	POLICY / PLAN #	DOCUMENT LOCATION

COMPANY		
CONTACT		
TEL / FAX / EMAIL		
DESCRIPTION	POLICY / PLAN #	DOCUMENT LOCATION

Form 10: Valuable Personal Assets

ITEM DESCRIPTION	LOCATION	BENEFICIARY

Form 11: Real Estate Assets

TYPE OF PROPERTY	
ADDRESS	
OWNER(S)	
FORM OF OWNERSHIP	
DEED LOCATION	
MORTGAGE COMPANY	
MORTGAGE REF. #	
TEL / FAX / EMAIL	
CONTACT	

TYPE OF PROPERTY	
ADDRESS	
OWNER(S)	
FORM OF OWNERSHIP	
DEED LOCATION	
MORTGAGE COMPANY	
MORTGAGE REF. #	
TEL / FAX / EMAIL	
CONTACT	

Form 12: Bills to be Paid

DESCRIPTION	ACCOUNT #	CONTACT INFO	AMOUNT	DUE DATE

Form 13: Assets and Liabilities Checklist

The following checklist provides an overview of some of the assets (what you own) and liabilities (what you owe) to think about when helping your loved one figure out their financial situation.

ASSETS	
Business interests	☐ Companies ☐ Corporations ☐ Partnerships
Cash	☐ Chequing accounts ☐ Savings accounts
Investments	**Short term:** ☐ Money market funds ☐ Treasury bills ☐ Short-term deposits **Long-term:** ☐ Bonds ☐ Mutual funds ☐ Property / real estate ☐ Stocks ☐ Term deposits
Life insurance	☐ Cash value if you ended the policy (not the death benefits)
Personal assets	☐ Art / antiques / collectibles ☐ Furnishings ☐ Jewellery ☐ Residence ☐ Vacation property ☐ Vehicles (cars, boats, etc.)
Retirement funds	☐ Employer pension plan ☐ Government pension plan ☐ Registered retirement savings plan

LIABILITIES	
Credit cards	☐ Bank credit card ☐ Store credit card
Loans	☐ Home mortgage ☐ Investment loan ☐ Life insurance borrowings ☐ Line of credit ☐ Student loan ☐ Vehicle loan
Miscellaneous	☐ Household bills (hydro, cable, etc.) ☐ Taxes (property, income, etc.)

Form 14: Calculating Net Worth

1. ASSETS: AVAILABLE CASH	ESTIMATED CURRENT VALUE
Cash (bank accounts – cheqing, savings)	
Short-term investments:	
Money market funds	
Short-term deposits	
Treasury bills	
Cash value of life insurance	
Other available cash assets:	
a.	
b.	
TOTAL: AVAILABLE CASH	
2. ASSETS: INVESTMENTS	**ESTIMATED CURRENT VALUE**
Business interests:	
Companies	
Corporations	
Partnerships	
Long-term investments:	
Bonds	
Mutual funds	
Property / real estate	
Stocks	
Term deposits	
Retirement funds:	
Employer pension plan	
Government pension plan	
Registered retirement savings plan	
Other investments:	
a.	
b.	
TOTAL: INVESTMENTS	

3. ASSETS: PERSONAL	ESTIMATED CURRENT VALUE
Art / antiques / collectibles	
Furnishings	
Jewellery	
Residence	
Vacation property	
Vehicles (cars, boats, etc.)	
Other personal assets:	
a.	
b.	
TOTAL: PERSONAL ASSETS	
TOTAL: ASSETS	
Add the totals from available cash, investment assets and personal assets	

4. LIABILITIES	ESTIMATED CURRENT VALUE
Credit cards	
Bank credit cards	
Store credit cards	
Loans	
Home mortgage	
Investment loan	
Life insurance borrowings	
Line of credit	
Student loan	
Vehicle loan	
Miscellaneous	
Household bills	
Taxes	
Other monies owing:	
a.	
b.	
TOTAL: LIABILITIES	

NET WORTH CALCULATION	
TOTAL ASSETS	
LESS TOTAL LIABILITIES	
NET WORTH	
Calculate net worth by subtracting the total liabilities from the total assets	

Form 15: Pre-planning of Arrangements After Death

A	ARRANGEMENTS FOR THE BODY
☐	Burial (indicate requested burial location) ______________________
	Indicate clothing and jewellery to be worn, along with any personal items to be placed in the casket ______________________
☐	Cremation (indicate where ashes should be scattered, buried or preserved) ______________________
☐	Yes, there is a pacemaker or metal implant (describe implant) ______________________
☐	No, there are no implants
☐	Organ or body donation (indicate what arrangements have been made and where the relevant papers are located) ______________________ ______________________

B	TYPE OF SERVICE
☐ Funeral ☐ Memorial ☐ Committal ☐ No service	
☐ Other ______________________	

C	LOCATION OF SERVICE
☐	Church or temple ________________
☐	Funeral home ________________
☐	Other ________________
D	**MUSIC TO BE PLAYED OR SUNG**
	List the hymns, chants, songs or other music to be included in the service. Include the names of any preferred singers or musicians.
	1. ________________
	2. ________________
	3. ________________
E	**READINGS**
	List favourite scriptures, readings, poems, etc. to be read during the service. Include the names of any preferred readers.
	1. ________________
	2. ________________
	3. ________________
F	**EULOGY**
	Identify the names of preferred people to deliver the eulogy.
	1. ________________
	2. ________________
G	**FLOWERS AND DONATIONS**
☐	Flowers appreciated for immediate family.
☐	No flowers please. Monetary donations appreciated for:
	1. ________________
	2. ________________
	3. ________________

H	PRE-PLANNING ARRANGEMENTS
☐	Yes, pre-planning arrangements have been made (identify memorial society or funeral home and location of paperwork): ____________________ ____________________
☐	No arrangements have been made.
I	**OTHER INSTRUCTIONS OR INFORMATION**
	____________________ ____________________ ____________________ ____________________ ____________________ ____________________ ____________________

Form 16: Phone Call Log

DATE	NAME	PHONE NUMBER	MESSAGE

Form 17: Estimating Funeral Costs

Professional Service Fees	
Funeral director and staff	$
Optional Services	
Embalming / cremation	$
Other preparations of the body	$
Viewing / wake service - facility and staff fee	$
Funeral / memorial service - facility and staff fee	$
Cemetery / graveside service	$
Hearse	$
Limousine	$
Casket / cremation urn	$
Burial plot / urn vault	$
Memorial / headstone	$
Cash Disbursements	
Floral arrangements	$
Catering	$
Musician	$
Other	$
TOTAL	**$**

Form 18: Planning a Service

LOCATION	
Address:	______________________
Contact:	______________________
Tel / Fax / Email:	______________________
Date / Time:	______________________
Seating capacity:	______________________
OFFICIANT	
Name:	______________________
Tel / Fax / Email:	______________________
MUSIC	
Before the service:	______________________
During the service:	______________________
	______________________
After the service:	______________________
Musician:	______________________
Tel / Fax / Email:	______________________
READINGS	
Poem:	______________________
Scripture:	______________________
Quotation:	______________________
EULOGY	
Delivered by:	______________________
Tel / Fax / Email:	______________________

FLOWERS	
Flower shop:	
Tel / Fax / Email:	
Flowers requested:	

PHOTOGRAPHS / MEMORIAL	
Photos:	
Memorial:	
Placement:	

MEMORIAL KEEPSAKE	
Format:	
Photo:	
Content:	

DONATIONS	
Charity:	
How to donate:	
Contact Info:	

GUEST REGISTER	
Type of register:	
Register attendant:	
Tel / Fax / Email:	

USHERS / GREETERS	
Name:	______________________
Tel / Fax / Email:	______________________
Name:	______________________
Tel / Fax / Email:	______________________
RECEPTION	
Location:	______________________
Catering contact:	______________________
Tel / Fax / Email:	______________________

Form 19: Writing an Obituary

The following outline can be used for writing an obituary.

Opening paragraph

Contains basic information such as the person's full name, date and place of death, and age.

Next of kin

Acknowledges surviving family members and important relationships.

Life overview

Includes highlights and accomplishments of the person's life, such as their occupation, education, special achievements, volunteer work, military service, special interests, hobbies or awards.

Funeral arrangements

Identifies funeral or memorial service arrangements, including information on any requests for charitable donations in lieu of flowers.

Form 20: Accounts / Organizations Checklist

The following form provides a list of some of the organizations that may need to be contacted after death.

Associations / Affiliations	☐ Alumni associations ☐ Automobile associations ☐ Business associations ☐ Frequent flyer programs ☐ Military associations ☐ Professional associations
Credit Cards	☐ Bank credit cards ☐ Gas station credit cards ☐ Store credit cards
Employment	☐ Employer ☐ Union
Government Offices	☐ Driver's licence ☐ Employment insurance ☐ Family benefits ☐ Income security / social security / social insurance ☐ Medical services plan / Medicare ☐ Land titles registry ☐ Pension / superannuation plan ☐ Post office, e.g., mail forwarding ☐ Taxation office ☐ Veterans affairs
Financial Institutions	☐ Banks ☐ Credit unions ☐ Investment companies / financial advisors ☐ Mortgage companies ☐ Stock brokers ☐ Trust companies
Healthcare Providers	☐ Chiropractor ☐ Dentist ☐ Doctors ☐ Optometrist ☐ Pharmacist ☐ Physiotherapist

Insurance Companies	☐ Automobile insurance ☐ Dental insurance ☐ Extended health insurance ☐ House insurance ☐ Life insurance ☐ Vehicle insurance
Memberships / Season's Passes	☐ Arts events, e.g., ballet, symphony ☐ Health and athletic clubs ☐ Mail-order clubs, e.g., music, DVDs ☐ Monthly home deliveries, e.g., wine club, vitamins ☐ Museums ☐ Public library ☐ Rotary, Kiwanis, Lions, Veterans' organizations and clubs ☐ Sports events, e.g., football, baseball
Social Networking Sites	☐ Facebook ☐ LinkedIn ☐ Twitter
Subscriptions	☐ Journals ☐ Magazines ☐ Newspapers
Utilities	☐ Alarm company ☐ Cable / satellite TV ☐ City services, e.g., garbage collection ☐ Electricity authority ☐ Gas supply company ☐ Internet provider ☐ Security service ☐ Telephone service

Form 21: Sample Death Notification Letter

TO WHOM IT MAY CONCERN

I wish to notify you of the death of:

Mr/Mrs/Miss/Ms

____
SURNAME

____
GIVEN NAMES

____
DATE OF BIRTH

____
STREET NAME / NUMBER

____
PROVINCE / STATE POSTAL / ZIP CODE

____
DATE OF DEATH

I understand the above-named person had dealings with your organization. The reference / membership / client number for your organization was ______________________________. Please amend your records accordingly.

If you need to contact me for further information, my name is ______________________________. I can be reached by phone at ______________________________.

____
SIGNATURE

____
ADDRESS

____
RELATIONSHIP TO THE DECEASED

____
DATE

APPENDIX 1: MEDICAL SPECIALISTS

SPECIALIST	AREAS OF EXPERTISE
Anaesthesiologist, or anesthetist	Anaesthesia (drugs that block the feeling of pain during surgery) and the medical care of patients before, during and after surgery.
Cardiologist	Heart and major blood vessels of the chest.
Endocrinologist	Endocrine system (endocrine glands and hormones) and associated diseases, including diabetes and thyroid diseases.
Gerontologist	Function and diseases of the aging patient.
Gynaecologist	Female reproductive organs.
Hematologist	Blood, the blood-forming organs and diseases of the blood.
Hepatologist	Liver, gall bladder, pancreas and biliary tract diseases such as hepatitis.
Immunologist	Immune system and related body defences, including the diagnosis of allergies.
Nephrologist	Kidneys.
Neurologist	Central nervous system, peripheral nervous system, and spinal column diseases.
Oncologist	Cancer and different treatment specialities, such as chemotherapy, surgery and radiation.
Ophthalmologist	Eyes and related visual pathways.
Orthopaedic doctor	Muscular system, the human skeleton and associated diseases, including arthritis and cerebral palsy.
Otolaryngologist	Ear, nose and throat disorders.
Palliative care specialist	Pain and symptom relief and emotional support in patients with terminal illnesses.

SPECIALIST	AREAS OF EXPERTISE
Pathologist	The study of disease through the analysis of tissue and body fluids.
Pediatrician	Infants, children and adolescents.
Pulmonologist	Lungs and the respiratory system, including diseases such as emphysema.
Proctologist	Rectum, anus and colon.
Psychiatrist	Emotional and behavioural disorders such as substance abuse, mental illnesses, dementia, depression and cognitive changes after a stroke.
Radiologist	Radiation used in medical imaging (e.g., X-rays), and the diagnosis and treatment of diseases.
Rheumatologist	Joints and other organ systems for diseases such as arthritis.
Urologist	Urinary tracts of males and females, and the male reproductive system.

APPENDIX 2

READING LIST – TALKING WITH CHILDREN ABOUT DEATH AND DYING

Bosak, Susan V. with Laurie McGaw. *Something to Remember Me By: An Illustrated Story for Young and Old*. Ontario: The Communication Project, 1997.

The true story of a grandmother and her granddaughter and how their relationship grows and changes over the years along with the memories they share.

Brown, Laurie Krasny and Marc Brown. *When Dinosaurs Die: A Guide to Understanding Death*. Boston: Little, Brown. 1996.

A book that explains in simple language the feelings people may have regarding the death of a loved one and the ways to honour the memory of someone who has died.

Buscaglia, L. *The Fall of Freddie the Leaf*. New York: Holt, Rinehart & Winston, 1983.

A story that uses nature and the changing seasons of life to explain how death can be seen as a natural part of living.

Mellonie, Bryan and Robert Ingpen. *Lifetimes: The Beautiful Way to Explain Death to Children*. New York: Bantam Books, 1983.

A book that talks about plants, animals and people to help children understand beginnings and endings.

Silverman, Janis. *Help Me Say Goodbye: Activities for Helping Kids Cope When a Special Person Dies*. Minneapolis, MN: Fairview Press, 1999.

An art therapy and activity book for children coping with death. Children are encouraged to express in pictures what they are incapable of expressing in words.

Stickney, Doris. *Water Bugs & Dragonflies: Explaining Death to Young Children. Revised.* Cleveland, Ohio: The Pilgrim Press, 2004.

The life cycle of water bugs and dragonflies helps children understand death.

Thomas, Pat and Leslie Harker. *I Miss You: A First Look at Death*. Hauppauge, New York: Barron's Educational Series Inc., 2001.

A book that talks about feelings and invites children to talk about how they're feeling.

MEMORIAL SOCIETIES IN CANADA

Memorial societies are organizations that inform and educate consumers on arrangements after death, and provide access to simple, affordable services through contracted funeral service providers. Membership in these organizations must be purchased before death.

British Columbia

Memorial Society of British Columbia (Provincial Office)

205 - 640 West Broadway
Vancouver BC, V5Z 1G4

Tel: 604-733-7705
Fax: 604-733-7730
Toll Free: 1-888-816-5902
Fax: 1-888-816-5903

Email: mail@memsoc.org
www.memsoc.org

Manitoba

Funeral Planning and Memorial Society of Manitoba

c/o 613 St. Mary's Road.
Winnipeg MB, R2M 3L8

Tel: 204-452-7999

funeralsocietymb.org

Northern Ontario

Memorial Society of Northern Ontario

PO Box 1355 Stn B
Sudbury ON, P3E 5K4

Tel: 705-671-3753
(24 hrs. answering service)

Email: msno@canoemail.com
www.memorialsociety.ca

Ontario

Federation of Ontario Memorial Societies Funeral Consumers' Alliance

55 St. Phillips Road
Etobicoke ON, M9P 2N8

www.myfuneralplan.org

Saskatchewan

Memorial Society of Saskatchewan

P.O. Box 1846
Saskatoon SK, S7K 3S2

Tel: 1-866-283-2677
(within the province only)
Tel: 306-374-5190

www.famss.ca

APPENDIX 4

NATIONAL / INTERNATIONAL PALLIATIVE CARE ORGANIZATIONS

Palliative care organizations are committed to enhancing quality of life for the terminally ill and to developing understanding and improved access to hospice and palliative care.

Canada

Canadian Hospice Palliative Care Association

A national organization advocating for quality end-of-life care in Canada, with a focus on public policy, public education and awareness.

www.chpca.net/Home

Europe

European Association for Palliative Care

A non-governmental organization recognized by the Council of Europe, which strives to develop and promote palliative care in Europe through information, education and research.

www.eapcnet.eu

International

International Association for Hospice and Palliative care

A non-profit organization helping to advance hospice and palliative care programs, education, research and favourable policies around the world.

www.hospicecare.com

United States

The National Hospice and Palliative Care Organization

The largest non-profit membership organization in the United States representing hospice and palliative care programs and professionals.

www.nhpco.org/templates/1/homepage.cfm

APPENDIX 5

CANADIAN PROVINCIAL PALLIATIVE CARE ORGANIZATIONS

Alberta

Alberta Hospice Palliative Care Association

ahpca.ca

Tel: 403-206-9958

British Columbia

BC Hospice Palliative Care Association

www.hospicebc.org

Tel: 1-877-410-6297

Manitoba

Hospice and Palliative Care Manitoba

www.manitobahospice.ca

Tel: 1-800-539-0295

New Brunswick

New Brunswick Hospice Palliative Care Association

www.nbhpca-aspnb.ca

Newfoundland and Labrador

Newfoundland and Labrador Palliative Care Association

Tel: 709-777-5742

Nova Scotia

Nova Scotia Hospice Palliative Care Association

www.nshpca.ca

Tel: 902-893-7171

Ontario

Hospice Association of Ontario

www.hospice.on.ca

Tel: 1-800-349-3111

Ontario Palliative Care Association

www.ontariopalliativecare.org

Tel: 1-888-379-6666

Quebec

Réseau de soins palliatifs du Québec

aqsp.org

Tel: 514-282-3808

GLOSSARY OF TERMS

Administrator	A person appointed by a court to handle the estate of a deceased person if there is no will, or if the will does not name an executor. An administrator is often the spouse, common-law partner or next of kin.
Advance directive	Advance decisions or instructions given by a person describing what actions should be taken for their health if they are unable to make those decisions due to physical or mental incapacity.
Anticipatory grief	Deep emotional distress that can occur when someone has been diagnosed with a life-threatening illness and death is expected.
Assets	Anything a person owns that has value. It includes tangible (i.e., physical) assets such as cars, property and jewellery, as well as intangible (i.e., cannot be physically touched) assets such as patents and trademarks.
Beneficiary	Any person or organization that is to receive funds or other property from an estate, a trust, or an insurance policy.
Bequeath	To give an item of personal property to a beneficiary after death by means of a will.
Bereavement	The state of being deprived of something or someone; a period of mourning and grief following the loss or death of a beloved person or animal.
Biopsy	The surgical removal of a sample of tissue from a living person for examination.
Burial	The placing of human remains in the ground, usually in a churchyard or cemetery.
Capital gain	A capital gain is the increase in value of an asset between the time it is bought and the time it is sold. A tax on capital gains commonly applies to the sale of assets like cottages, stocks and bonds, as well as land, buildings or equipment used in a business.

Capital loss	A capital loss is the decrease in value of an asset between the time it is bought and the time it is sold.
Capital property	Any property that, if sold, would result in a capital gain or a capital loss. Common types of capital property include cottages, securities such as stocks and bonds, land, buildings, and equipment used in a business or rental operation.
Catheter	A tube put into the bladder so urine can drain into a specially designed collecting bag. Sometimes used when a person is no longer able to control their bladder.
Certified death certificate	A legalized copy of an original death certificate that is usually required for settling an estate, including insurance policies and death benefits.
Clearance certificate	A certificate issued by a federal government tax authority certifying that all amounts owed by the deceased have been paid. It is recommended that the executor of an estate obtain a clearance certificate before distributing assets to ensure that the executor does not become liable for any amounts owed by the deceased.
Columbarium	A niche, chamber or wall designed for storing urns containing cremated remains.
Committal service	A ceremony that takes place at the graveside or where the ashes of a deceased person are to be buried. The service itself may involve the lowering of a casket into the ground, the placing of remains in a tomb or vault, or the burying of cremation ashes.
Coroner	A public official responsible for investigating deaths, particularly deaths that happen suddenly or under unusual circumstances, and determining the cause of death.
Creditor	A person or entity to whom a debt is owed.

Cremation	A process that uses intense heat to reduce a body to bone fragments, which are then crushed or ground into ashes.
Death	The permanent ending of all vital functions of the body including the heartbeat, brain activity and breathing.
Death certificate	A permanent legal record of the fact of death of an individual issued by a government official such as a registrar of vital statistics. A death certificate provides important information, such as an individual's full name, gender, date of death, place of death, place of birth, place of residence, registration number and date of registration. An official death certificate or certified copy is needed for dealing with the will and settling the estate.
Death registration	The process of officially registering a death with the appropriate government organization such as the vital records and registration office of the local public health department. Once the death has been registered, a formal death certificate can be issued.
Deceased	A person who has died.
Designated beneficiary	A person or organization named in a will or life insurance policy to receive property or other benefit payments when the owner dies.
Do not resuscitate order	A legal document instructing medical professionals not to perform lifesaving measures if a person's heart stops or if they stop breathing.
Embalming	The process of treating a dead body with a preservative substance to stop decay and prepare the body for burial.
End of life care	Healthcare and support services for dying people and their families.

Enduring power of attorney	A legal document that authorizes someone else to carry out decisions and manage financial and most legal decisions on behalf of a loved one, even in the event of physical or mental incapacity.
Estate	The assets or items a person owns at death, such as real estate or jewellery, as well as the personal debts or liabilities owed. The distribution of an estate is documented in a will.
Estate planning	Advance planning for the administration and distribution of an estate upon the death of the owner.
Estate taxes	A tax imposed on an estate in some jurisdictions.
Eulogy	A speech given during a funeral or memorial service in honour of a person who died.
Executor	A person or trust company appointed in a will to administer the estate and carry out the wishes of a person who died.
Executrix	A female executor.
Funeral service	A ceremony to commemorate the life of a deceased person, often held with the body or cremated remains of the deceased person present.
Funeral director	A licensed professional who supervises and/or prepares the final arrangements for a deceased person's body and oversees all funeral preparations. It is common practice for a funeral director to complete the death registration process.
Graded benefit life insurance	A type of life insurance designed to provide coverage for the person's "whole life." A percentage of the death benefit is paid out if death should occur in year one of the policy, with a larger percentage becoming available in each subsequent year.

Grief	Great sadness or intense sorrow, especially at the death of a loved one.
Hospice	A specialized healthcare facility that looks after people who need care at the end stage of a terminal illness.
Hospice care	Holistic care provided in a specialized facility for people at the end stage of a terminal illness; often associated with community programs.
Incontinence	Lack of control of the bowels or bladder.
Interment	The act or ceremony of placing the body of a dead person in a grave.
Intestate	Describes a person who dies without leaving a legally valid will.
Intestacy rules	Local statutory rules governing what happens to an estate if there is no will.
Inurnment	The placement of cremated remains in an urn, which is then placed in a niche, crypt, grave or other location in a cemetery.
Legal representative	An executor, administrator or liquidator responsible for settling the estate of a deceased person.
Liabilities	Debts owed by a person including credit card balances, unpaid bills, taxes, mortgages, etc.
Life insurance	Life insurance is a legal contract between a policy owner and an insurance company that guarantees a specific sum of money to be paid to a designated beneficiary upon the death of the insured.
Liquid assets	Assets that can be converted into cash quickly and easily.
Liquidator	The role of the liquidator is similar to an executor if there is a will. For estates without a will, the liquidator acts as the administrator of the estate. In Quebec, the distribution of assets for all estates is undertaken by a liquidator.

Living will	A legal document that describes a person's wishes to have or to forego medical treatments that prolong or sustain life in the event that a person is not able to speak for themselves.
Medical certificate of death	A document signed by a doctor or coroner identifying the date, location and cause of a person's death.
Memorial service	A ceremony to commemorate the life of a deceased person generally held without the body or remains present, allowing more flexibility around the timing of the service.
Morgue	A room or building where dead bodies are kept.
Named beneficiary	A person or organization named in a will or life insurance policy that will receive property or other benefit payments when the owner dies. When a specific beneficiary is named in a life insurance policy, the proceeds of the policy will not be subject to the will or to probate and will pass directly to the named beneficiary.
Net worth	The amount by which a person's assets (what they own) exceeds their liabilities (what they owe).
Niche	A space in a columbarium used for the inurnment of cremated human remains.
Notarized	A document carrying the authenticated signature of a person required or authorized to sign it, such as a notary public.
Notary public	An individual legally empowered to officially witness signatures on documents, certify the validity of a document, collect sworn statements and administer oaths.
Obituary	A notice or announcement of a person's death.
Officiant	A person responsible for planning and leading a funeral, memorial or committal service.

Organ donation	An advance directive donating a person's organs or tissues after death for transplantation or research.
Palliative	Treatment focused on providing relief from the symptoms, pain and stress of a serious illness without effecting a cure.
Palliative care	Healthcare to relieve suffering and improve the quality of life for people with a serious illness. Addresses not only physical pain, but also emotional, social and spiritual suffering.
Pathology	The branch of medicine dealing with the nature of disease, especially changes in body tissues and organs.
Power of attorney	A legal document authorizing a person to carry out decisions and manage affairs on behalf of someone else. A power of attorney automatically ceases to be valid when a person is no longer mentally or physically capable to manage their affairs
Premiums	The amount owing for the purchase of insurance coverage, paid as a lump sum or by instalments.
Probate	Probate refers to the legal process of reviewing a will to prove that it is valid and authentic, and to confirm the authority of the executor named in the will.
Promession	An ecologically-conscious method for disposing of human remains by freeze drying the body, reducing it to a fine powder which decomposes naturally.
Proof of death	An original, notarized or certified true copy of a death or burial certificate.
Statutory rules	The written laws of a jurisdiction.
Terminal illness	An advanced stage of a disease that cannot be cured or treated, and is ultimately considered fatal.

Testament	A legal document that describes how a person wants their assets distributed upon death. Another name for a will.
Testator	A person who has signed a will expressing their wishes for what they want to happen with their assets upon death.
Trustee	A person named in a will to administer an estate and carry out the wishes of the person who died, for the benefit of the beneficiaries named in the will.
Viewing	A special gathering for family and friends to allow for the viewing of the body of a recently deceased person. A viewing may take place several days in advance of a funeral or memorial service in a funeral home, a family home or at a church. Sometimes used interchangeably with the term wake.
Wake	A special gathering for family and friends to allow for the viewing of the body of a recently deceased person. Traditionally, a wake is held the night before a funeral or memorial service, often in the home of the deceased. Sometimes used interchangeably with the term viewing.
Will	A legal document that describes how a person wants their assets distributed upon death, and identifies a person or organization responsible for carrying out their wishes.
Whole life insurance	A type of life insurance designed to provide coverage for the person's "whole life" rather than a specified term. The premiums cover the insurance risk along with a savings or investment component that increases in value over time.

BIBLIOGRAPHY

Berlin, Rebecca. *What Is a Living Will?* Available at: www.alllaw.com/articles/wills_and_trusts/article7.asp

Callanan, Maggie. *Final Journeys: A Practical Guide for Bringing Care and Comfort at the End of Life.* New York, New York: Bantam Dell, March 2009.

Canadian Bar Association. *Power of Attorney and Representation Agreements.* July 2012. Available at: www.cba.org/BC/public_media/wills/180.aspx

Canada Revenue Agency. *Preparing Returns for Deceased Persons 2012.* Available at: www.cra-arc.gc.ca/E/pub/tg/t4011/t4011-12e.pdf

Canadian Life and Health Insurance Association Inc. *A guide to life insurance.* March 2009. Available at: www.clhia.ca/download/brochures/Brochure_Guide_To_Life_ENG.pdf

Cochrane, Michael G. *Canadian Real Estate Law: Forms of Ownership.* Insomniac Press, 2007. Available at: www.mycanadianrealestatelaw.com/formsofownership.html

Deloitte & Touche. *Canadian Guide to Personal Financial Management.* Scarborough, Ontario: Prentice Hall Canada Inc., 1997.

Duhaime, Lloyd. *Duhaime's Legal Dictionary.* Available at: www.duhaime.org/LegalDictionary.aspx

Dyer, Kirsti. *Helping Children Cope with Death.* Available at: journeyofhearts.org/grief/kids_death.html

Fayerman, Pamela. *What are patient navigators?* The Vancouver Sun, Feb 25/11. Available at: www.vancouversun.com/health/What+patient+navigators/4305467/story.html

Foster, Sandra E. *You can't take it with you: the Common-Sense Guide to Estate Planning for Canadians; Third edition.* Etobicoke, ON: John Wiley & Sons Canada Limited, 2000.

Fraser, Kathleen. *When I'm Gone: Practical Notes for Those You Leave Behind.* Erin, Ontario: Boston Mills Press, 2009.

Harris, Darcy L. and Howard R. Winokuer. *Principles and practice of grief counseling.* New York, New York: Springer Publishing Company, LLC, 2016.

James, John W. and Russell Friedman. *When Children Grieve: for Adults to Help Children Deal with Death, Divorce, Pet Loss, Moving, and Other Losses.* New York, New York: HarperCollins Publishers, 2001.

Kessler, David. *The Needs of the Dying: A Guide for Bringing Hope, Comfort, and Love to Life's Final Chapter.* New York, NY: Harper, 2007.

Kübler-Ross, Elisabeth and David Kessler. *On Grief and Grieving: Finding the Meaning of Grief Through the Five Stages of Loss.* New York, NY: Scribner, 2005.

Kuhl, Dr. David. *Facing Death, Embracing Life: Understanding What Dying People Want*. Doubleday Canada, Ltd., 2006.

Kuhl, Dr. David. *What Dying People Want: Practical Wisdom for the End of Life.* Canada: Anchor Canada, 2003.

Macmillan, Karen . . . [et al.] *A Caregiver's Guide: A Handbook About End-of-life Care*. Ottawa, Ontario: Transcontinental Printing, 2004.

Mayo Clinic. *End of Life: Caring for a Dying Loved One.* Available at: www.mayoclinic.com/health/cancer/CA00048

Mungall, Constance. *Probate Guide for British Columbia*. Canada: International Self-Counsel Press Ltd., 1997.

Noel, Brook and Pamela D. Blair. *I Wasn't Ready to Say Goodbye: surviving, coping & healing after the sudden death of a loved one.* Naperville, Illinois: Sourcebooks, Inc., 2008.

Noel, Brook and Pamela D. Blair. *I Wasn't Ready to Say Goodbye: a companion workbook for surviving, coping, & healing after the sudden death of a loved one.* . Naperville, Illinois: Sourcebooks, Inc., 2008.

Noel, Brook. *The Physical and Emotional Effects of Grief*. Available at: funeralplan.com/griefsupport/griefsteps.html

Ray, M. Catherine. *I'm With You Now: A guide through incurable illness for patients, families, and friends.* Bantam Books, 1997.

Royal Bank of Canada Booklet. *Settling an estate.* RBC Financial Group, 2002.

Tapp-McDougall, Caroline. *The Complete Canadian Eldercare Guide: Expert Solutions to Help You Make the Best Decisions for Your Loved Ones.* Mississauga, ON: John Wiley & Sons Canada Ltd, 2004.

INDEX

S

T

U

V

W